How To Get Your Legs Higher in a Développé Devant

Written by Lisa Howell

Disclaimer

The contents of this manual, including text, graphics, images, and other material are for informational purposes only, and is provided as an accompaniment to the online video course. Nothing contained in this manual is or should be considered or used as a substitute for professional medical or health advice, diagnosis, or treatment. The information provided in this report is provided on an "as is" basis, without any warranty, express or implied.

Never disregard medical advice from any treating doctor or other qualified health care provider or delay seeking advice because of something you have read in this document. We urge that dancers seek the advice of a physician or other qualified health professional with any questions they may have regarding a medical or health condition. In case of emergency, please call your doctor immediately.

The Ballet Blog holds no liability or responsibility for any injury or complication that may arise from following this information. Any use of this manual is voluntary and at your own risk. If you require further information about any injury, please feel free to contact us to organise an individual consultation either in person or via Skype/Phone.

Published 2019 by The Ballet Blog

© Copyright The Ballet Blog 2019

ALL RIGHTS RESERVED

Except for the purpose of fair reviewing, no part of this publication may be reproduced or transmitted in any form or by any means, electronic or mechanical, including photocopying, recording or any information storage and retrieval system, without prior written permission from the publisher.

Contents

Introduction	5
Assessing Range	11
Turnout Devant	12
Hamstrings in all Positions	14
6D Breathing	16
Mobilise	19
Thoracic Mobilisers	20
Hip Flexor Mobilisers	24
Tucks and Tilts Sequence	25
Trigger Point Releases with a Ball	27
Cupping for Upper and Lower Legs	28
Hamstring Mobilisation Sequence	30
Isolate	33
4 Point Sit Backs	34
Cushion Squeezes	35
QF Heel Squeeze	36
Iliacus Suck - in Lying	38
Psoas Activation in 4 Point	40
Turnout with Foot on the Wall	41
Integrate	43
Waiter Bow	44
Cushion Squeezes with Leg Extension and Rotation	45
4 Point Turnout with Endurance	46
Cushion Squeezes with Oblique Curl	47
Standing Iliacus Suck	48
Adult Crawling Sequence	49
Function	53
QF Transfer with Port De Bras	54
Développé Devant in Lying	55
Placement at the Barre, with Fondu and Rise	57
Adage in Class	59
Putting Together Your Program	60

Introduction
Welcome to the Program

Welcome to this unique program which will teach you how to get your legs higher in your adage, especially in a développé devant, as part of our Training Turnout series. To get the most out of this course, make sure you purchase the online video component through our online portal www.theballetblog.com.

Dancers all over world constantly ask us about how they can get their legs higher and the secrets to this are sometimes a little bit different than they realise. Many people think that if they apply resistance or put weights on their legs and just practice the movement then it will get better. Unfortunately, that often results in more load through the hips, increased tension, more restriction and frustratingly slow progress.

So, what we do in this program is a little different.

But rather than take my word for it I wanted Jessi Seymour, our beautiful model for this program, to talk about what she experienced when working through the program. Jessie is a stunning dancer, but she was having trouble supporting her extensions to the front. She had been doing the program for just two weeks when the videos were filmed, and I asked her to give a little bit of feedback about what changed since she started working on this very specific set of exercises.

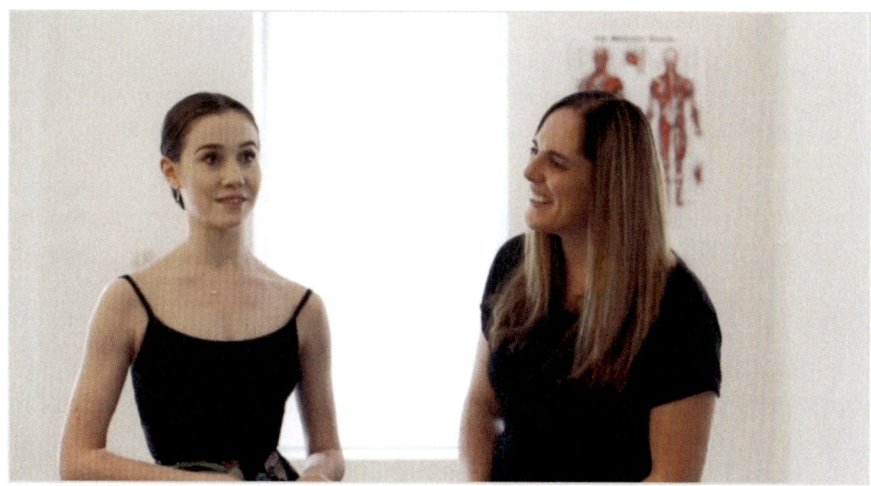

"A big thing that has changed is it feels ten times easier! I never knew it could be that easy, with that little effort to get my leg up and feel so in control, without using so much muscle. Using the least amount of effort to get the nicest line is really amazing! I've never felt like that before."

Jessi Seymour - Dancer

How to Work Through the Program

In order to get the most out of this program, please resist the desire to skip to the end and do all of the higher level work first. Please make sure you that you go through all of the videos in sequence, because this will give you a real understanding of all the foundations that need to be developed to support your extensions. It also helps if you have done our standing leg turnout sequence first, as everything needs to be built on a solid base, so if you haven't done any work on your supporting leg please do so.

The first thing you need to learn in regards to your extensions is understanding the anatomy of the hips, and then how to assess your hips in detail, to determine what range of motion you actually have. A big mistake that a lot of dancers make is that they are trying to have their extensions higher than their available flexibility. If you are struggling with your flexibility, you may want to have a look at our Front Splits Fast program or some of our other fascial mobilisation techniques available online, to ensure you have the range to be able to place the leg where you want it to be. If you're pulling up against resistance all the time your extensions are always going to feel difficult.

In this program I utilise a strategic training process that I use whenever I am working on improving any kind of technique.

1. **Mobilise:**
It is important to mobilise all of the areas that we need to be nice and free to allow an effortless développé. This helps hydrate the tissues in preparation for activity and is also a time to check in on how mobile you are feeling on any particular day as this can vary.

2. **Isolate:**
Isolation is about making sure the deep stabilisers in the spine, the pelvis and around the hip are all actually working. Sometimes a weakness in just one of these essential muscles can make a real difference to your long term performance, and can result in excessive loading of other muscles.

3. **Integrate:**
Integration is where you start to use the deepest, stabilising muscles combined with some of the more superficial movement muscles, so that they all work together as a team. This is an essential stage in reprogramming your movement patterns to transform your dancing.

4. **Function:**
Functional exercises teach you how to build this new coordination of the muscles around the hip into the end movement of your développé devant, so that you can perform it effortlessly in class and on stage.

Anatomy of the Hip & Spine

Before we start the program it helps if you understand a little bit about the anatomy of the hip, pelvis and spine, and their mechanics during movement. This will help you understand why it just doesn't make sense to add more resistance to your hip flexors if you want to flex the hip, because that may sound like a good idea! There is a really interesting setup in the anatomy of the spine and its relationship to the hip and pelvis that took me many years to work out in relation to getting your legs higher in a développé devant and á la seconde. I want to go through this so that you have a good understanding of why we need to be so specific with the exercises before you start working on the program.

The biggest complaint that most people have when trying to hold the leg en l'air is that they feel jamming in the top of the hip and gripping in the thigh. A lot of dancers say:

> *"My teacher tells me not to use my thigh muscles,*
> *but I don't know how to use anything else!"*

Once you understand the relationship of the stability in your low back to your pelvis and the deep control in the hip, this makes a lot more sense.

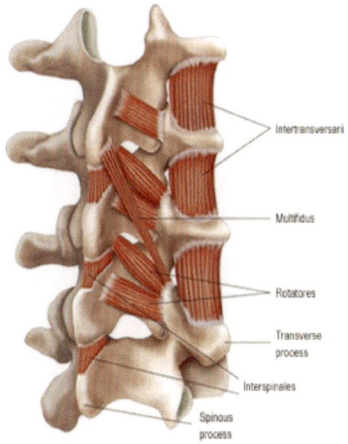

Deep Spinal Stabilisers

Very close to the spine are some tiny, deep stabilising muscles called Multifidus, Rotatores, Intertransversarii, and Interspinalis. These small muscles are designed as dynamic, segmental stabilisers of the spine and are responsible for the movement of one vertebrae on the next. They are designed for endurance, so can work at low intensity for long periods of time. They also help support the action of the ligaments, so are even more important in hypermobile individuals with lax ligaments and very mobile backs.

Erector Spinae and QL

You also have several bigger back muscles in a group called the Erector Spinae, which includes your Iliocostalis, Longissimus and Spinalis muscle groups. These are longer, thicker muscles that attach into multiple vertebrae and are more designed for power and movement, so get fatigued easily. You have a Longissimus and a Spinalis muscle in both the Cervical and Thoracic Spine.

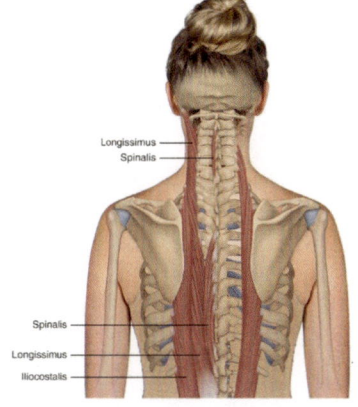

Hip Flexors

The Psoas Major muscle is a deep hip flexor which attaches to the front of the spine and has a role in stabilising the spine. It arises from the spine, and then comes forward to the front of the hip, attaching to the upper, inner aspect of the thigh bone, which allows it to act as a hip flexor. One of the normal functions of Psoas Major is to help stabilise the spine, however normal people don't ask their leg to be above their head for most of the day.

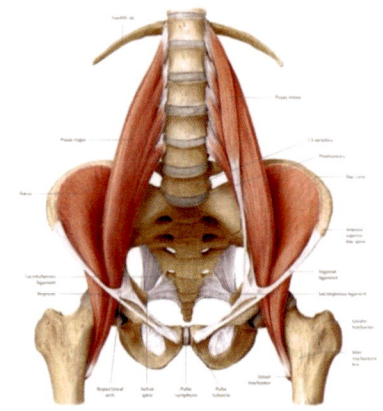

If you are a dancer, and you are wanting to use your Psoas Major more as a hip flexor (to support your extensions) you can not rely on it so much as a spinal stabiliser.

To have effective hip flexion above 90 degrees you need to train the deep back stabilisers to be more effective in stabilising the spine. This in turn allows the Psoas Major to reduce its spinal stabilising role in order to be able to work more effectively as a hip flexor. Weak spinal stabilisers result in a chronically tight Psoas Major. This is the reason why we discourage deep sustained stretches or hands on "releases" of Psoas. If it is tight, it is usually tight for a reason, and this reason must be addressed. If the Psoas Major is forcefully released it may make the spine unstable. Improved spinal stability will allow Psoas Major to release naturally.

The second muscle that joins with Psoas Major to make the Iliopsoas Tendon is the Iliacus, which attaches to the inside of the pelvis. Ideally, Iliacus works subtly to centralise the hip, allowing Psoas Major to flex the hip. If the hip is centralised correctly, then the load of the leg is controlled from much deeper and doesn't get transferred to the more superficial hip flexors such as your TFL and your Rectus Femoris.

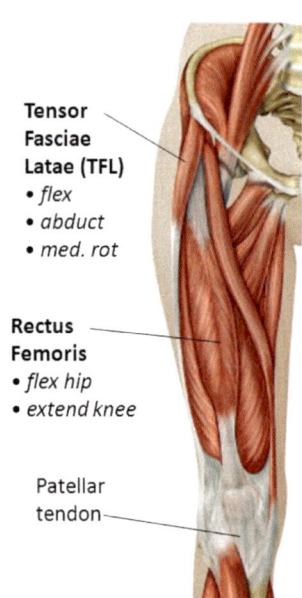

Therefore, if a dancer is complaining that they're struggling with the height of their extensions, or are experiencing gripping in their hips or in the front of their quads during adage, the first thing I do is look at the stability of the spine, and the centralisation of the hip in the socket.

How do I know if my spine is unstable?

You can identify if your spine is not very stable if you have one or more of the following:

- You feel like you need a massage in your low back all the time
- You tend to sit with the low back slightly flexed
- You tend to get a sore back when you are sitting or standing for long periods of time
- You feel restricted into a forward bend or into a back bend
- You crack your back every day (or multiple times a day)
- It's hard to maintain a good sitting position.

These are all signs that you are using your big back muscles a little bit too much and you may need to look at ways to improve your stability in the deeper layers.

We are going to put a lot of focus on this in this program because the more stable you are through the lower back the lighter and easier your extensions will become.

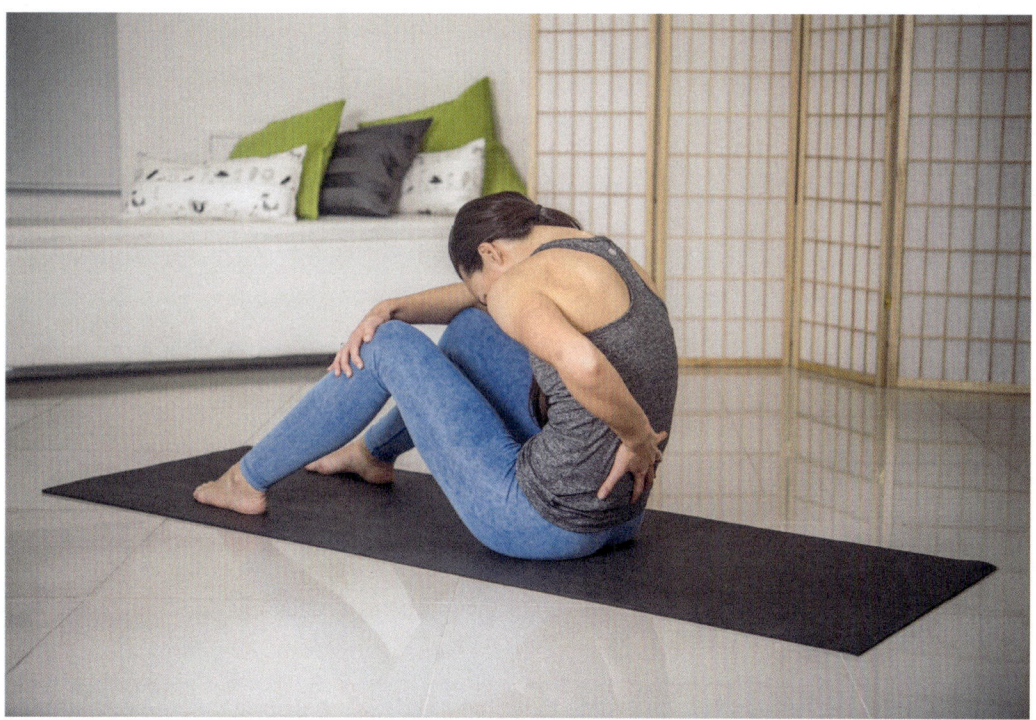

Notes:

Assessing Range

The first stage of the program is assessing your current range to see how much you have to work with. Spending time working on these specific areas of mobility will help allow your leg to be placed with ease in your extensions. This program is great if you've already got the flexibility to mount your leg easily to the front but you're struggling to hold your leg devant. If you don't have much mobility, it's very important to work on that first, as if you're fighting against resistance it's going to create a lot more tension around your hips.

You will need a partner to help with these tests so that you can focus on relaxing as much as possible. If you are working with your arms to try to test your own leg, you may get an inaccurate reading.

Make sure to note your findings from each test in the chart on each page. Noting down the quality of the restriction is important as this give you a lot of information about how to improve your range.

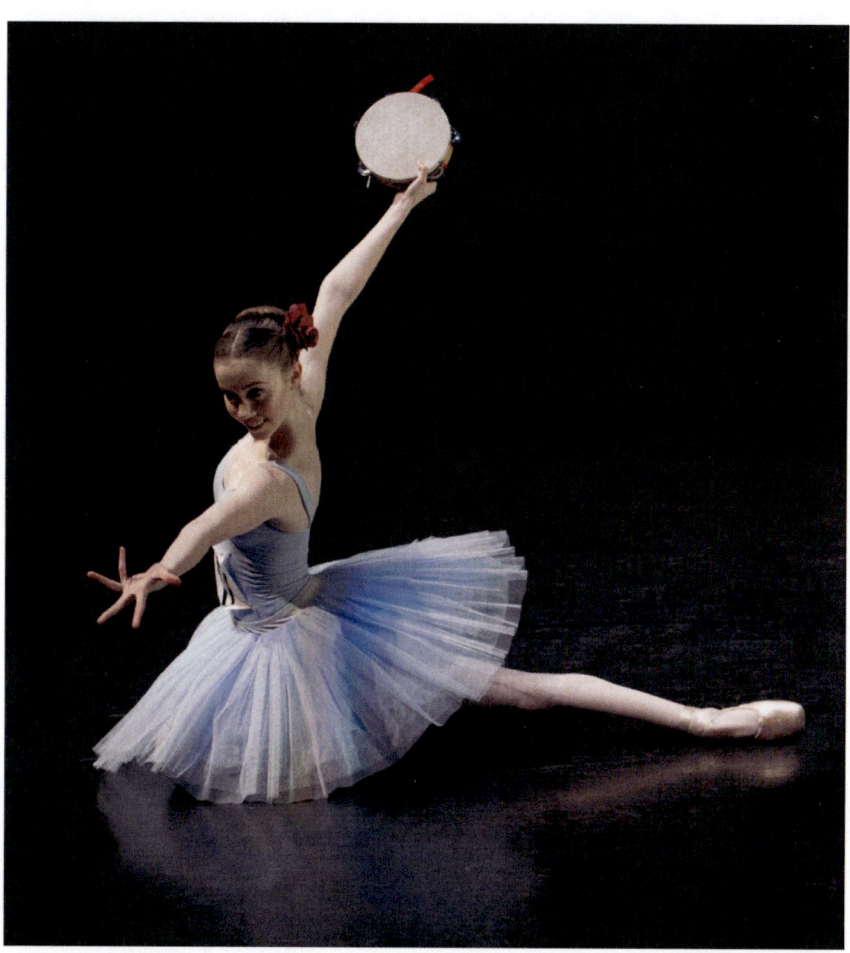

Turnout Devant

The first thing we want to do is have a look at your turnout range devant and your flexibility to the front. Interestingly, many dancers have far more range than they are aware of in this position. The more you can rotate the leg in this position the easier it is to rotate the quads to the side, allowing the deeper hip flexors and inner thighs to support the weight of the leg when working devant.

1. Start lying on your back on a yoga mat. Try to relax completely as your partner lifts your leg to flex both the hip and the knee to 90 degrees.

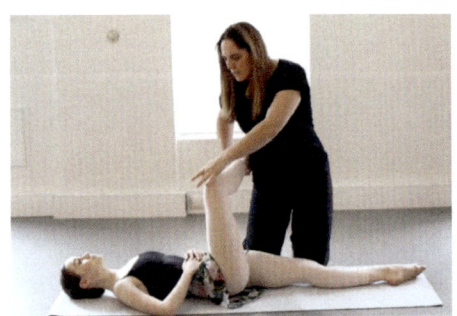

2. Ensure that the thigh bone is vertical, and the hips are square. Place your fingertips on your hip bones to monitor your own pelvic position.

3. The assessor gently rotates the lower leg, keeping the upper leg vertical, until either of you start to feel a little bit of resistance, but before the pelvis starts to move. Make sure that there is no strain in the knee.

4. Note where in your body you feel pulling or what stops your hip from rotating further, and ask the assessor to estimate your range. If the starting position is 0 degrees, and having the shin bone parallel to your waist is 90 degrees, ask the assessor to estimate your range.

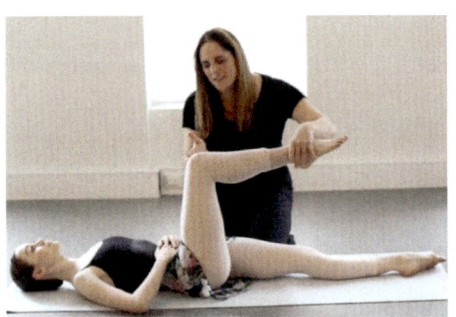

5. Aim for above 45 degrees in this position on both sides before moving forward with the higher levels of the program. Some dancers will easily have this range, others may have to spend a few weeks working on their range before this is possible.

6. Repeat the assessment on the other side. As long as there is a nice muscular stretch and you have decent range, then you should be able to continue with the program. If you are markedly restricted, or there is pain or blocking in the front of the hip, then this should be worked on before starting the strengthening exercises in the program.

Test	Left	Right
Turnout Devant		

Becoming aware of the location and quality of the restriction will give you lots of information about how best to improve your range. Use the chart below to establish a strategy for improving range, and consult the appendix at the back of the book for more details on specific releases if needed.

Location and Quality of Restriction	Likely Structure	Suggested Release Techniques
A pulling or stretch on the outer hip	Muscular or fascial tension around Piriformis or Gluteus Medius	Tennis ball releases for Gluteus Medius and Piriformis Cupping for outer hip, Lateral Line Mobiliser, Pigeon Pose.
Pinching or sharp pain in the front of the hip	Thickening in the capsule or Iliopsoas Tendon. Possible Labral Tear. Do not push into this as it will aggravate it.	Consult Health Professional for accurate diagnosis. Focus on postural control - not sitting into hips. Iliacus suck exercises to recentre hip. Gentle Hip Flexor mobilisers - avoid direct stretches at the site of pain.
Pulling into the hamstring or inner thigh	Fascial tension or over use of the hamstrings for turnout.	Hamstring Mobilisers Cupping for hamstrings Sub-Occipital Release
No feeling of restriction, it just stops	Bony block or very tight posterior capsule.	Tennis ball releases for Obturator Internus and Piriformis Internal rotation stretch

Notes:
_____
_____
_____
_____
_____
_____
_____
_____

Hamstrings in all Positions

Next you need to assess your hamstrings. Everyone is a little different, and we can also be quite different day to day, so even if you normally have fantastic range please go through this test carefully to see what subtleties you can feel. It is also important to make sure that you assess the hamstrings in both parallel and in turnout, as a lot of dancers are markedly restricted when they rotate the leg fully due to a fascial wind up down the back of the leg.

1. Start by lying on your back on a mat, with your pelvis square and spine in neutral

2. Lift your leg up into parallel, making sure your hips are nice and square. If you are quite mobile you can do this yourself, however if you struggle to get the leg past 90 degrees, it will be easier to get someone else to test your leg for you.

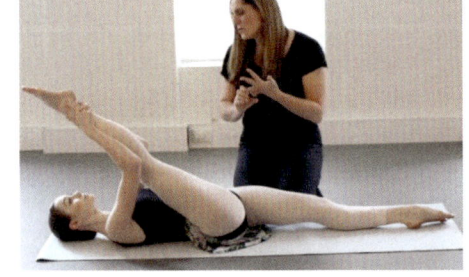

3. Try to keep your back in neutral, rather than flattening it to the floor, and make sure the opposite foot and leg are relaxed on the floor.

4. Note the position in range where the restriction starts to come on, and also the placement and quality of the restriction. Is it a sudden grab in the middle of your hamstrings? Or possibly a long line of pull behind the knee? Some dancers may feel a deep pulling right up by their sitting bone.

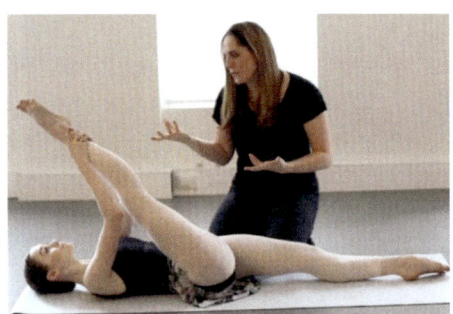

5. Next, turn the leg out and place it where you'd like your Développé Devant to be. Some people have a lot of range in parallel yet when they turn it out they feel much more restricted. You want to make sure that you have good range in turnout to be able to nicely place your leg in your adage.

6. Relax the leg back down and repeat on the other side. Note your results in the box below, and then check for the possible solutions to any restriction in the table on the following page.

Test	Left	Right
Hamstrings in Parallel		
Hamstrings in Turnout		

Location and Quality of Restriction	Likely Structure	Suggested Release Technique
One point of muscular pulling in the middle of the hamstring	Muscular tension in the hamstrings	Gentle muscular stretch when warm Cupping Technique Trigger point releases in the muscle belly
More spread out tension over a bigger area on the back of the leg	Fascial Tension in the superficial back line	Hamstring mobilisers Cupping techniques Ensure adequate hydration
Strong pull or possible pain at the top of the hamstrings/ sitting bone	Hamstring insertion or Tendinopathy	Eccentric loading of hamstring muscles Avoid stretching Focus on subtle activation of the deep back muscles and pelvic stability
A distinct line of pull down the back of the leg, calf or behind the knee	Neural Tension	Tennis ball releases for piriformis Deep calf mobilisers Foot massage techniques Tucks and tilts series for back mobility 6D breathing for rib mobility

After reading through the suggestions above and including any other exercises you know from other programs, note down the exercises, mobilisers and stretches that you need to do to improve your mobility in these tests. Also note down any ideas of how you can fit these into your current weekly program.

Notes:

_____
_____
_____
_____
_____
_____
_____
_____
_____
_____
_____
_____

6D Breathing

Most people don't realise the importance of breathing correctly or they haven't really thought about how much it may be affecting their dancing. When I bring up breathing with a lot of dancers they say, "Oh I know I don't breathe well!" but they haven't actually thought of looking into ways of actually improving it. The first part of the 6D breathing exercise is all about assessing what is actually happening, when you breathe, and on getting all parts of the lungs correctly involved. We then need to learn to use the breath to facilitate a gentle "collecting" of the inner unit as the base for your deep core control. The importance of this in relation to your développé devant comes from the stability component. If the core stabilisers, including the Pelvic Floor, Tranversus Abdominis, the Diaphragm and the deep back muscles (Multifidus, Rotatores, Intertransversarri etc) are dynamically working, this allows Psoas Major to be more available to lift the leg en lair.

Set Up
Start lying on your back with your knees bent and feet flat on the floor. Ensure you're in a neutral spine, with the front of the pelvis in a horizontal position (not a flat back) and check to make sure your big back muscles are relaxed by feeling them with your fingertips. Some dancers may need to use a folded up towel to support the low back in this position in the beginning to allow the big back muscles to release. If you have any pain in your back or your hips, try resting your calves on a chair, but use a towel to support the back in neutral.

1. Front and Back - Place one hand over the diaphragm and the other hand around the back of the rib cage. Close your eyes and focus on your natural breathing. See if you can feel how much movement happens at the front of the ribcage compared to the back and determine the percentage in each direction. I.e. 90% front to 10% in the back, or 70% to 30%. A lot of people will feel that it is very imbalanced to the front, and very little coming to the back initially.

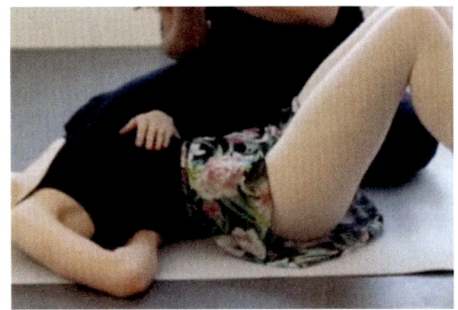

If you feel that it is imbalanced, try to correct it using your mind. Keeping your eyes closed, see if you can imagine a little more air coming into the back of the lungs. If this is effective, wonderful! If this is still difficult it may mean that there is more of a mechanical restriction and you need to do some more fascial mobilisers to loosen the tissue to allow a more natural breathing pattern.

2. Side To Side - Place your hands on the sides of your rib cage, up quite high so you're hands aren't down near your waist. With normal, natural breathing, compare the movement of the right side of the rib cage to the left in terms of both volume and speed. A lot of people will find that they have a lot more movement on one side compared to the other. This can be due to having a small scoliosis, or may simply be due to sleeping on one side the night before.

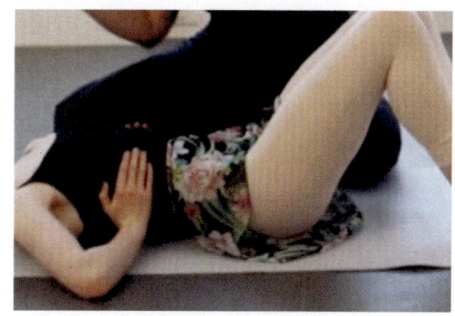

Notice again whether any imbalances can be corrected simply by using your mind, or whether the restriction will need to be worked on when we progress to the mobilising exercises.

3. Up and Down - Place one hand on your neck and the other down on your low belly. Observe your breathing and note how much difference there is at the top compared to the bottom. This is the one test where we don't want to be balanced 50/50. You want to feel the majority of the movement down into your low abdomen. Make sure that your neck muscles and the upper chest stay relaxed. However, make sure that you are not using too much muscle power to push the stomach out and pull it in.

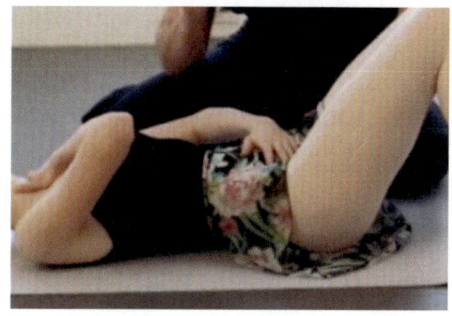

You want to use very little tension and just feel a gentle float and a fall of the abdomen.

4. Collecting the Core - Place your fingertips and thumb tips together to make a little triangle and place them on the low pelvis, below your navel. Combining all of the movements you've done, take a big breath in allowing the ribcage to expand forward and back, side to side, a little bit up but mostly down, expanding the whole abdomen. Exhale with a long "Shhhh" sound. Feel the low abdomen, pelvic floor and deep back gently "collect" as you exhale.

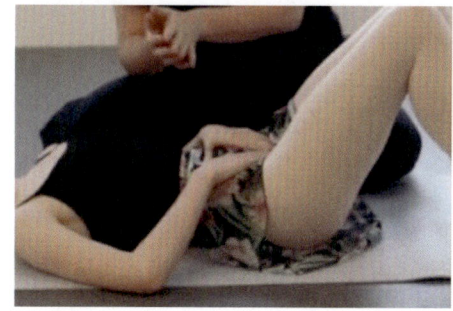

Repeat 3 - 4 times, extending the exhale for as long as possible, but without feeling any bracing in the outer abdomen or back muscles. Repeat this with normal breathing, without the sound, to feel a very gentle collection of your core with each breath. This allows you to train your deepest core muscles subtly and with every day activities.

Notes:

Mobilise

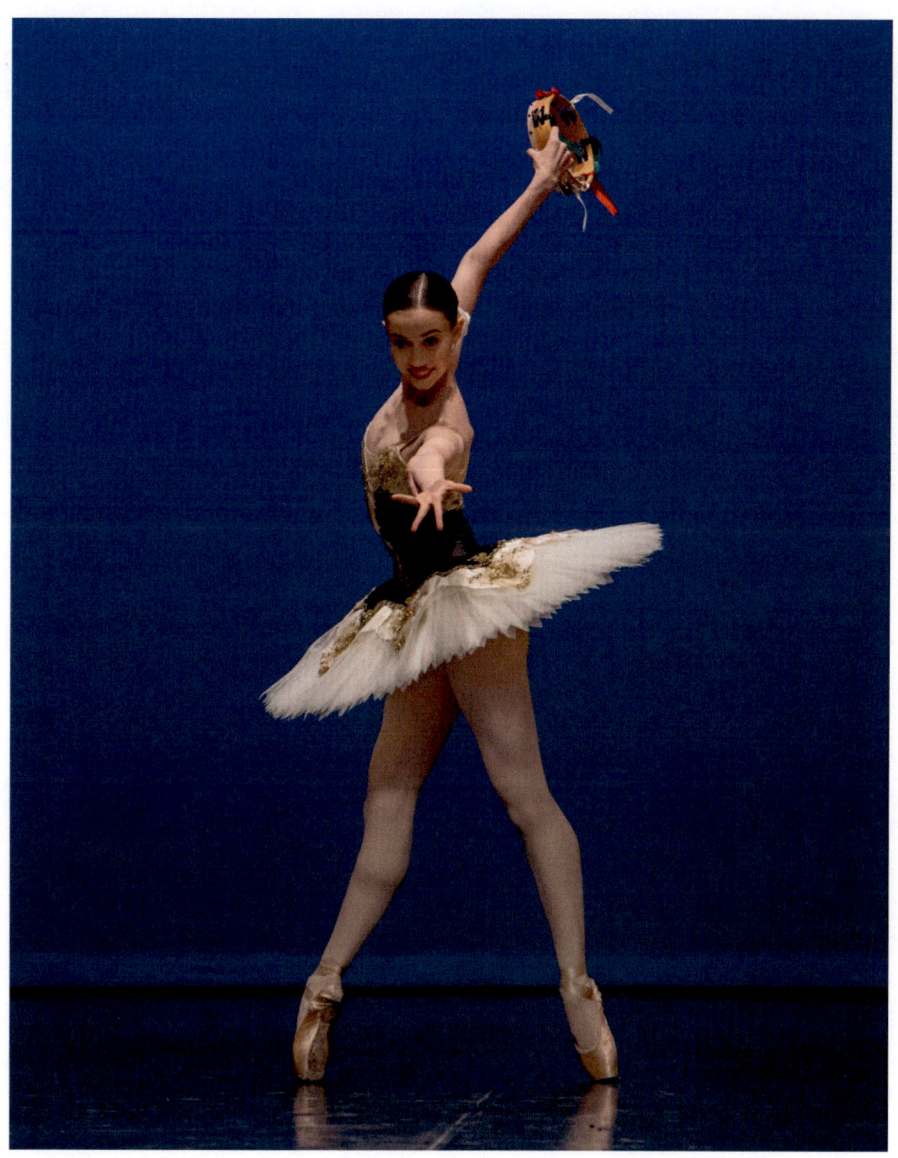

Mobilisation of the tissues that allow the leg to be beautifully placed is essential in getting the effortless float that we all desire in a développé devant. This section goes far beyond regular static stretching, which I usually consider to be the slowest and most dangerous way of attempting to get more flexible.

Even if you have fantastic range, I encourage you to incorporate the following mobilisation techniques into your training over the next few weeks, to open out your entire fascial system.

Thoracic Mobilisers

This Thoracic Mobilisation sequence is great for helping to free up the muscles and fascia around your ribcage to allow you to breathe a little more easily. It's also amazing how much this sequence affects your general flexibility into a forward bend, an arabesque, and especially the mobility of your hamstrings when mounting the leg to the front. This is due to its effect on all of the fascial lines in your body that cross the ribcage. This is a really nice set of exercises to use as part of your warm up before going into any dance class, and is also good to do in detail before you start moving onto the other parts of the program.

Note: If you feel any pulling or numbness into your hands with this exercise, this may indicate a restriction in the sliding of the nerves in your arms. Simply relax the wrist and elbow as you go into the reaches, but still perform the rib cage movements. If this is slow to resolve, we recommend consulting a local Physiotherapist or Osteopath who works with neural mobility issues to get some specific hands on treatment to help restore your range.

1. **Forward Reaches**

Start in a wide second position in parallel with your knees slightly bent. Reach forward with the right arm, feeling energy lengthening forward through your fingers, and also back through the opposite elbow, then repeat to the other side. While this may look like an upper body exercise, you also need to think about what is happening in the rest of your body as well.

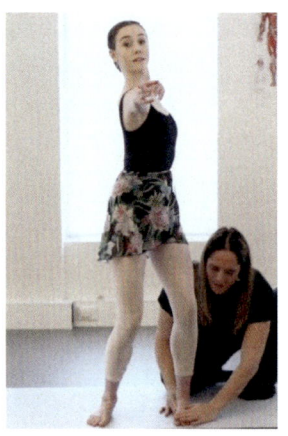

- Allow the ribcage and pelvis to rotate around a central axis, rather than leaning forward too much, and let this rotation spiral all the way down to the legs and feet.
- The same foot as the arm reaching forward will pronate (flatten/roll in), and the opposite foot will supinate (arch up).
- A lot of people are very rigid through their feet, so this might take some practise, and some dancers will need to do some gentle massage techniques to allow more foot mobility.
- Allowing the feet to move really helps make this a whole body mobilisation and can transform your flexibility in many areas.
- We suggest doing between 4-8 of these reaches in each direction. Keep focused on maintaining fluidity through the entire movement, rather than just hitting the end position.

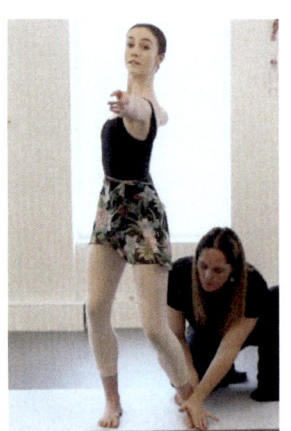

2. Upward Reaches

Place your left hand on your shoulder and reach the right arm up and over to the ceiling. Soften the right knee as the right arm reaches to the ceiling and let the pelvis tilt.

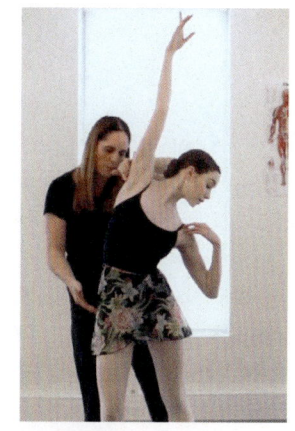

- You want to create the longest line between your armpit and hip, really lengthening out between your ribs.
- Some dancers really struggle with this at first, so if this is you, then practice the hip tilt on its own first, before adding the arm reach.

3. The Octopus

This variation creates a really lovely feeling of openness in one side of the ribcage, while compressing the other.

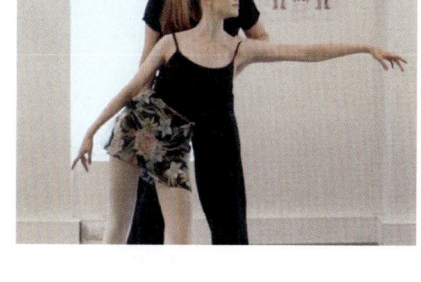

- Stand with the feet in a slightly wider second position.
- Shift the ribs off to the left and reach out with the left arm, reaching as far as you can towards the side wall.
- Keep a gentle awareness of your deep core, and try not to hyperextend the low back.
- If you feel any pain, discomfort or instability in the low or mid back, reduce the magnitude of the mobiliser, until you have been working on the exercises in the Isolation section for a few weeks.
- Repeat 8 times to each side, trying to soften 2mm deeper each time.

4. Backward Reaches

Reaching to the back can really help restore your rotation, and free up your thoracic spine. However, take care with this movement, as many people are very stiff in this direction due to the fact that they just don't do it on a regular basis!

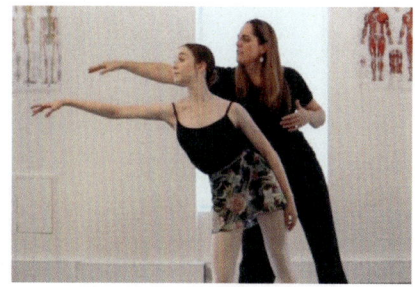

- Place your right fingertips on your right shoulder and reach for the back wall with your left hand, whilst reaching forward with the right elbow.
- Maintain softness in the knees and look back at your extended hand, allowing the right foot to pronate and the left foot to supinate.
- Try to spiral around a central axis, rather than going into a back bend.

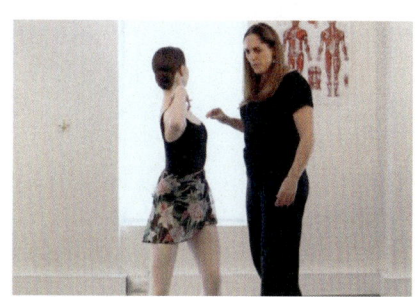

5. Spartacus

I like to call this exercise Spartacus, and always imagine Carlos Acosta performing for some reason!

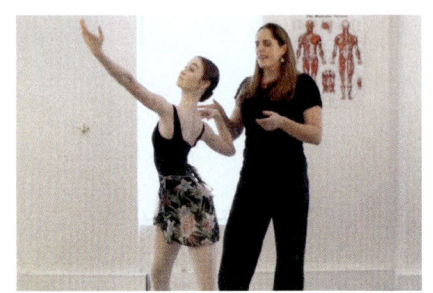

- Keep your right fingertips on the right shoulder, and sweep the left arm up to the top front corner of the room.
- Your arm should be angled at around 45 degrees up to the front,
- Feel equal energy down and back through the right elbow, as well as up and forward through the left hand to feel a nice spiral through the ribcage.

6. Shelf Reaches

Even more people are restricted in this direction, as most of us restrict our movement patterns to what is in front of us on a day to day basis.

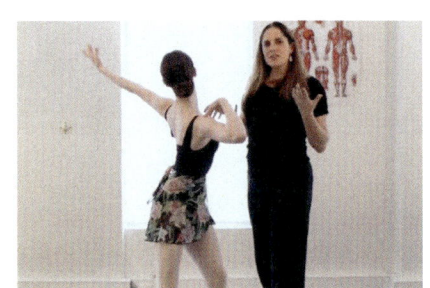

- With your left hand, reach back and up to the opposite back corner.
- This really helps open out the chest area, especially if you tend to breathe into the top of your chest, or spend too much time on your phone!

7. Flexed Forward Reach

You also can do a couple of different variations to mobilise all aspects of the head of the ribs.

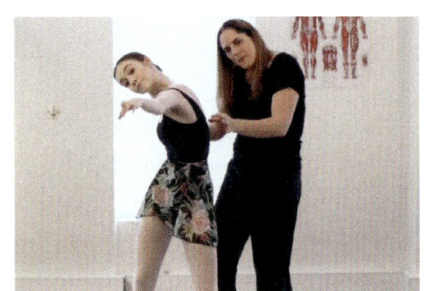

- Reach forward with the left arm and flex and rotate the ribcage a little. Really round out through the rib cage, breathing in to enhance the expansion in the back of the lungs.
- Repeat to the other side, really curling forward each time.

8. Extended Forward Reach

Finally, repeat the same forward reach with a little extension of the upper back.

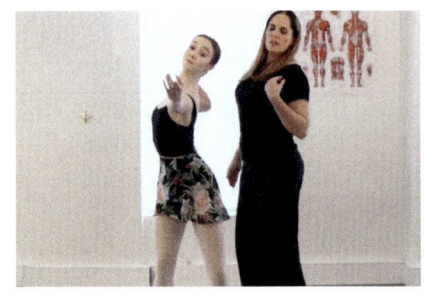

- This really helps to unwind all of the arm lines and the upper back.
- Aim to feel a high release in the upper back, rather than sinking into the low back.
- You should not feel any numbness or tingling into the hands or fingers.

9. Re-Assess your 6 D Breathing in Standing

After doing all of the mobilisers, notice whether it has made a difference to your mobility into a forward bend, the mobility of your rib cage and the ease at which you can breathe more deeply.

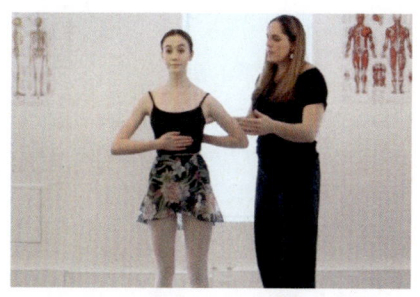

- Place one hand on the front of your ribcage, over the diaphragm, and one hand on the back of your rib cage.
- Close your eyes and compare your expansion front and back.
- Repeat the assessment from side to side feeling for evenness in volume and rate of expansion.
- Check your balance of movement in the neck and upper chest versus the lower belly.
- This is sometimes much harder to find in standing, so feel free to reassess in lying if this is easier.
- You'll often feel much more freedom in the rib cage after doing those exercises.
- Repeating the "Shhhhhh.." activation exercise in standing can help you to find your true core in a more functional position.

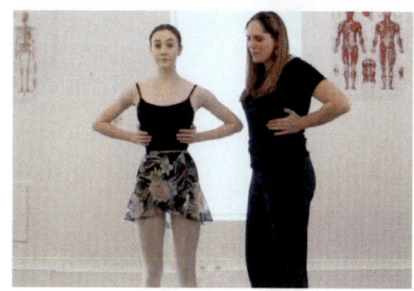

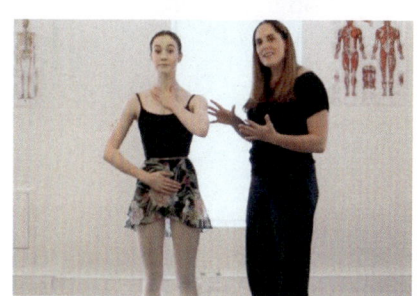

Notes:

_____
_____
_____
_____
_____
_____
_____
_____
_____
_____
_____
_____
_____

Hip Flexor Mobilisers

A lot of dancers do very strong hip flexor stretches especially if they are feeling tight in the hips, however strong static stretching can actually do more harm than good, by inhibiting and irritating the muscles you need to lift your legs to the front. These subtle hip flexor mobilisers are aimed at hydrating and mobilising the fascia rather than stretching the muscles and are a much better way to gently release tension and improve range in the front of the hip. The aim is to gently traction the tissues and release the stretch to allow fluid into the area. This helps lubricate and nourish the area, hydrating the fascia to make it more extensible.

Note: You never want to feel any sharp pain in the front of your hips. Aim for a slow, juicy mobiliser and a general awareness of lengthening in the tissues over an extended area, rather than a strong or painful stretch just in one place.

Starting Position
Place one foot forward and the other foot behind, keeping the body vertical. Stay high on your demi-pointe with the back foot, and place your hands on your hips. If you have any issues with the mobility of your big toe, you may place a folded towel under the back foot, under toes 2,3,4 and 5 to offload the big toe joint.

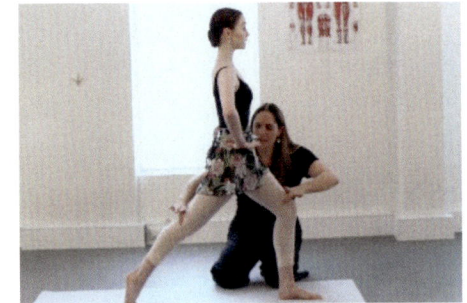

Basic Version:
Keeping the spine vertical gently press the heel back behind you and let the front knee come forward. This movement is more of a split than a lunge. You should start to feel a gentle opening in the front of the hip and upper thigh. Glide into position until you feel a subtle stretch and then back out of it. Keep the back knee straight, pelvis vertical, and focus on consciously opening the front of the hip. Do about 4 - 5 repetitions and then repeat on the other side.

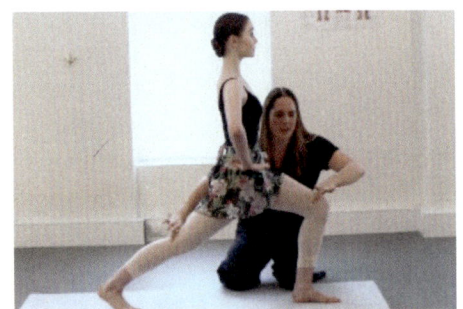

Arm Reach
Using the same placement as the first variation, glide into position, while simultaneously reaching up and over with the same arm as the back leg. Keep lifted through the front of the pelvis, but it is ok to let the hip of the rear leg drop a little to lengthen the side waist. Aim for a real reach, not a classical ballet arm for this exercise.

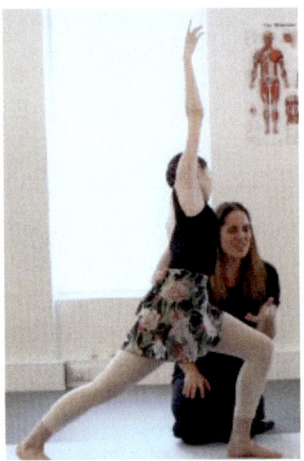

Tucks and Tilts Sequence

This Tucks and Tilts sequence really helps to develop subtle pelvic stability and spinal control. It's a great exercise to do when you warm up before class as it helps you restore optimal range of motion to your pelvis and spine before you start training. For example, if you've been doing a certain variation the day before that has lots of extensions you may be feeling a little tight when arching your back. If you've been doing a contemporary piece that is very flexion based you may be feeling more restricted in a different direction.

This exercise helps your brain connect with the muscles responsible for very subtle movements of your spine and pelvis. When performing any adage, you need to be able to subtly control your pelvis in multiple different directions. To explain this I often use the metaphor of learning a new language. When you learn a new language you'll usually learn simple words like hello, goodbye, yes, no, please and thank-you. As you become more articulate you begin to have more words in your vocabulary so you can explain what you want a little more. As you learn more subtle control of the pelvis you can give your pelvis much more subtle corrections you can be a lot more artistic with your gesture leg rather than being really rigid through the pelvis.

1. **Forward and Back**

- Start by placing your finger tips on the hip bones, making sure your back is in a neutral position and your big back muscles are off.
- Using as little muscle tension as possible, slowly roll the pelvis back so that the lower back flattens into the floor.
- Make sure that the front of the hips and the abdominals are relaxed.
- Then reverse the movement, arching the lower back.
- Note any points of tension and whether you are tighter in one direction.
- If there is a restriction in either direction, whether that is due to pain, stiffness or simply lack of control, use the opposite direction and movement to treat it. I.e. If there is restriction in extension (arching your back) go into flexion, and do 10 slow side to side movements with the pelvis.
- Then go back to the original movement to retest.
- Your aim is to be able to do ten slow movements forward and back with no pain

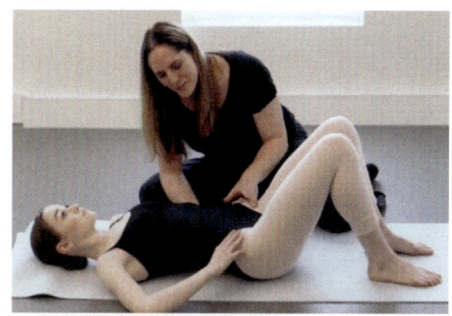
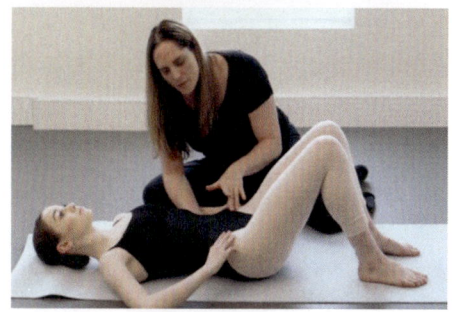
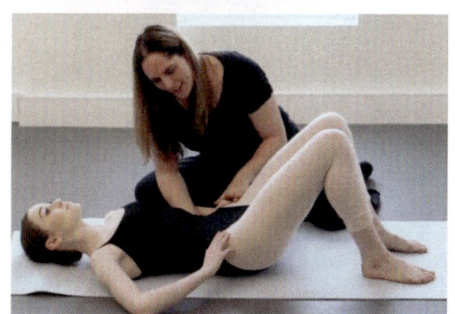

2. **Side To Side**

- Keeping the front of the pelvis horizontal with the floor, slowly pull the right hip up towards the right lower ribs. Focus on contracting the right side muscles and lengthening out the left side.
- Repeat on the left, noticing any restriction, pain or difficulties in coordinating the movement.
- If there is pain or restriction in lifting one side (i.e. right hip hitch), use the opposite direction (left hip hitch) and the opposite movement (flexion and extension / tuck and tilt) to fix it.

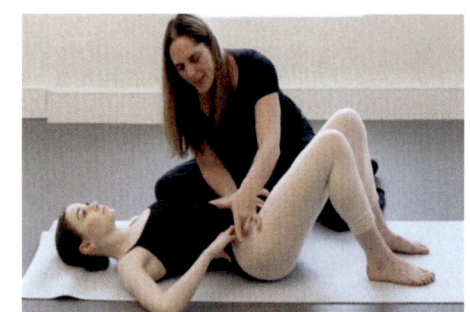

3. **Rotation**

- Try rotating the pelvis from side to side, by feeling one hip heavy and falling back to the floor, allowing the other to float to the ceiling
- Both knees should stay pointing at the ceiling.
- Often this movement is uncoordinated rather than painful so simply practice the movement slowly.
- However, if one side is markedly restricted compared to the other, and then use the opposite direction, opposite movement rule.

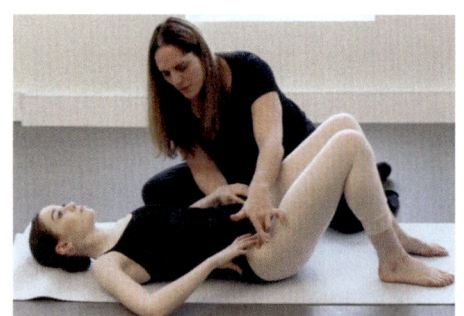

4. **Figure 8**

- Once you can perform all directions effectively without any pain or restriction, you can combine them all by moving the pelvis in a figure 8 movement.
- This movement may take a while to master, but it is an excellent way to get all of the small muscles in the low back and pelvis working naturally together.
- Start in neutral, feeling weight through the centre of the sacrum. Roll up the sacrum, flattening the low back to the floor. Rotate the pelvis to the right, feeling the point of pressure move over the top of the right buttock, then down the outer side of the buttocks, underneath the buttocks, to come to the tip of the sacrum with the back slightly arched. Roll up the sacrum and repeat to the left.
- Perform eight figure 8's in each direction.

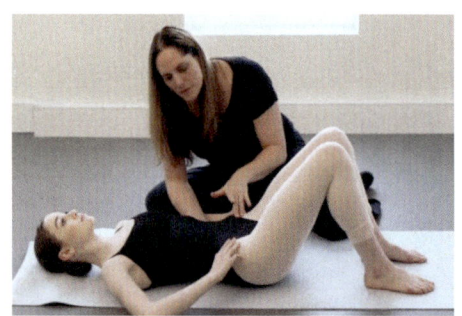

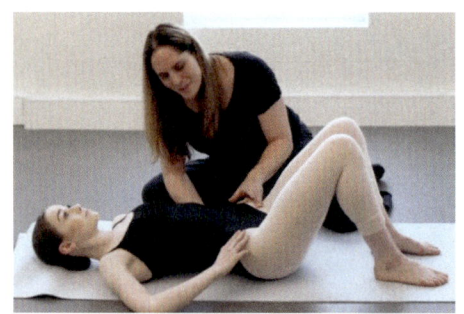

Trigger Point Releases with a Ball

Using a tennis ball to release trigger points in the Gluteals and Turnout Muscles can really help improve the mobility of your hamstrings and range into turnout, allowing the leg to be placed much more easily in your développé devant. Once you are aware of which muscles have increased tone you can use your conscious mind to deliberately relax the muscle you're working on.

- Start lying on your back with the feet flat to the floor, knees bent. Place the ball underneath one side of your pelvis, in the meaty part of your bottom. Place the other hand, held in a fist, under the other side of the pelvis to help keep it level

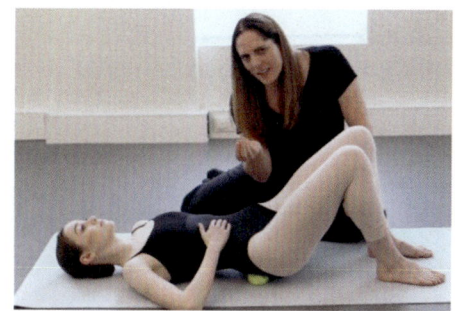

- Gently tuck and tilt the pelvis to find a tight point of tension ideally close to the point where you felt a stretch when testing turnout devant.

- Adjust your pressure until you feel about a 3/10 in intensity.

- Close your eyes and focus on breathing. As you breathe in experience the tension there and as you breathe out see if you can relax the whole bottom.

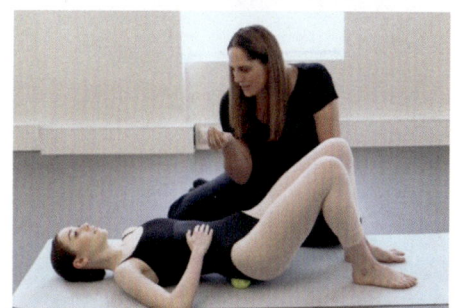

- If the sensation does not release, use less pressure.

- You don't want to feel any pins and needles coming down your leg, just a little muscle tension that you can release after 2-3 breaths.

- Keep in mind that this exercise is about internally letting go of your subconscious hold of that muscle, rather than massaging the muscle.

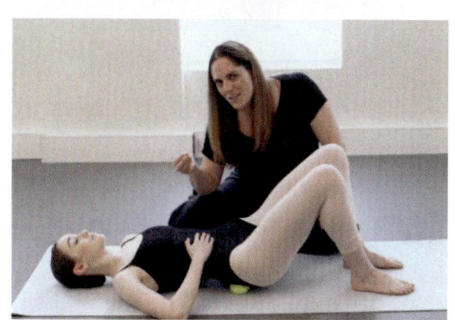

Note:
- This may take a bit of practice!
- You can try close to your tailbone or up and around the top of your buttocks.
- If you think of a nice rounded M shape from your tailbone up and over the buttocks.
- We suggest you buy a good quality branded tennis ball as the cheaper ones you buy from the dollar store often break when you sit on them.

Cupping for Upper and Lower Legs

Cupping is a great technique for helping mobilise and hydrate the layers of fascia in your upper and lower legs. This technique aims to traction out the layers of fascia, improving hydration, blood flow, extensibility and removing any adhesions between layers. This can be safely done by young dancers at home, and is a wonderful adjunct to their flexibility work. Many dancers find this a very effective way to release the tissues that are causing tension in their hips and legs, allowing you to lift your leg more easier in a développé devant.

What is Cupping? Cupping therapy has a long history of application in several asian cultures. Traditionally, a flammable substance, such as alcohol, herbs, or paper, is placed in a cup made of glass, metal, wood, or bamboo. The material inside the cup was set on fire to create a vacuum. As the fire goes out, the cup is placed upside down on the body in specific points to treat various health conditions according to traditional Chinese medicine. Cupping in this form often leaves large bruises on the skin.

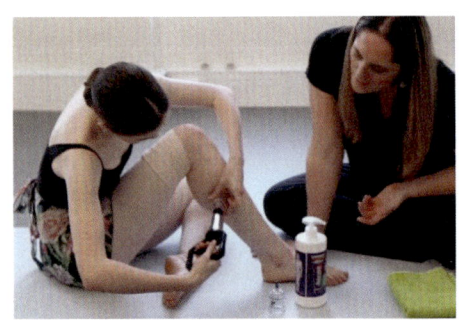

We use a totally different approach to cupping, which uses a plastic cup, and a small suction gun, to create a gentle vacuum inside the cup. Lotion is applied to the area to be treated, a small vacuum created, and then the cup is moved slowly and consistently up and down and across the fascial lines. There should never be any bruising after doing this technique.

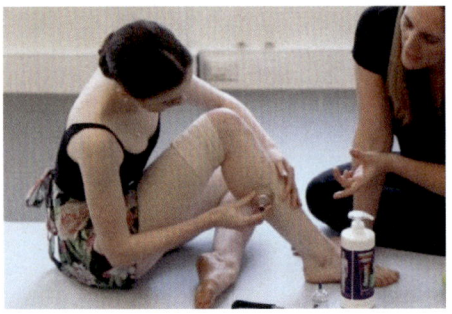

- Start with putting some massage cream on your leg.
- Place a cup on your leg and use a half squeeze of the cupping gun to gently create traction in the top layers of skin.
- The skin should never draw up past the lowest black lines on the cup, and always keep the cup mobile to avoid bruising.
- Move the cup gently up and down the leg, noting any areas of restriction where the cup moves more slowly.
- You should be able to move the cup easily with two fingers.
- Visualise fluid coming into area to create more space.
- Try working on the outer side of your lower legs, your hamstrings, quadriceps and the muscular parts of your hips and bottom.

Note:
- Tighter areas will cause the cup to move more slowly
- You don't want to leave marks on the skin. A slight redness might occur, this just means more blood is flowing to the area.
- It should feel like the tissues are loosening and freeing up as you work over an area.
- If it gets too tight take the cup off by lifting the little seal on the top and try again.
- You don't want to go over the back of the knee, neck or groin. Stick to bigger areas of muscles and avoid any visible blood vessels.
- You can use any cream; it just needs to be something that will allow the cup to slide and not absorb too quickly. Massage cream works well, but you can use olive oil at a pinch!

Notes:

Hamstring Mobilisation Sequence

The last mobiliser to do before getting started with all of the strengthening exercises is a Hamstring Mobilisation Sequence. These are not strong hamstring stretches, but are more dynamic mobilisers designed to increase hydration in all the tissues that surround the hamstrings. When doing these mobilisers, please make sure that the tension is felt around the back of the thigh, rather than down into the calf. If you do feel anything down in the calf, and especially if there is any sharpness or tingling to the quality of restriction, it may be a neural restriction rather than a fascial pull. If you do feel this, try going back to the trigger point releases through the bottom or more cupping along the back line or the base of the calf to release.

1. **Hamstring Mobilisers in Parallel**

- Start standing in parallel with your hands on your hips.
- Place one foot back, keeping both feet in parallel.
- Slowly fold at the hips, dropping the sit bones back to the wall behind you, bending the supporting leg, while keeping the front leg straight.
- Fold forward with the spine in neutral, keeping your hips square.
- Make sure not to flatten the low back, or overly arch the upper back
- You should feel a nice gentle stretch into back of the upper thigh.
- Once you have mastered the positioning of the spine, try deepening the mobiliser by reaching the arms forward in front of you, remembering to keep the hips square.

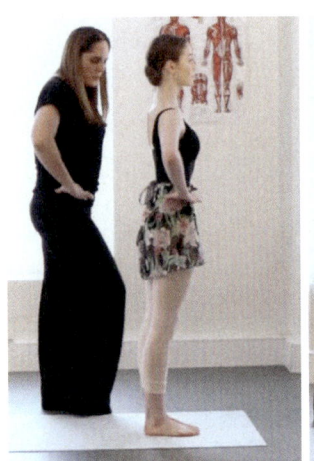
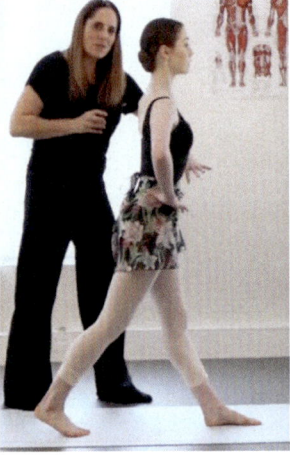
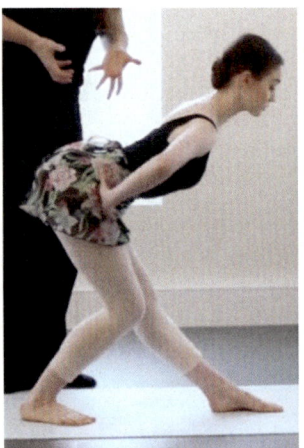
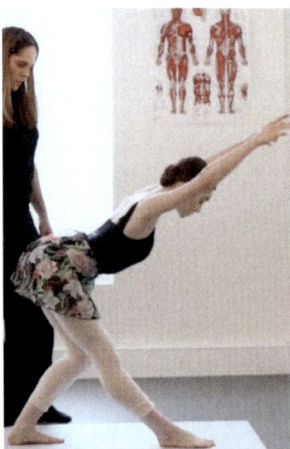

2. Turned Out

- Standing in first position, place one foot behind and drop the hips back, leaving the front foot in place.
- Try and keep the hips nice and square to the front, as it is very easy for them to twist in this variation.
- Remember to go just until the first point of restriction. You may not have as much range as you expect initially, but it will soon improve.
- This mobiliser helps improve your flexibility in rotation that you need for your extensions devant.

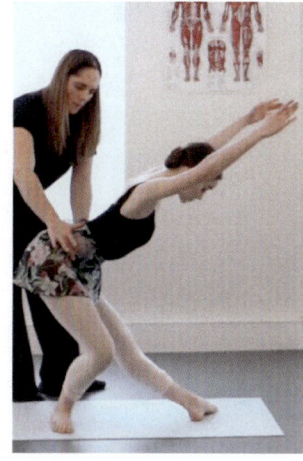

3. Turned In

- Start in standing with the feet turned in, in a 'pigeon toed' position.
- Step back with one leg as in the previous versions, keeping the hips square and leaning forward with the spine in neutral.
- This variation really helps target the medial hamstrings which are often neglected
- Repeat 8 times on each leg
- You should not feel any pain in the inside of the knee of the back leg. If you do, keep the back leg in parallel and just turn the front leg in.

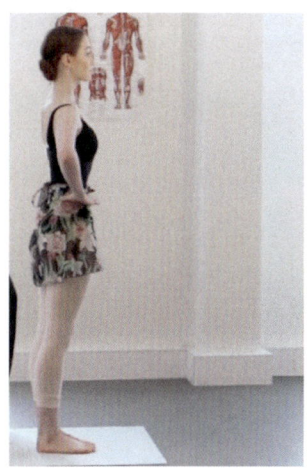 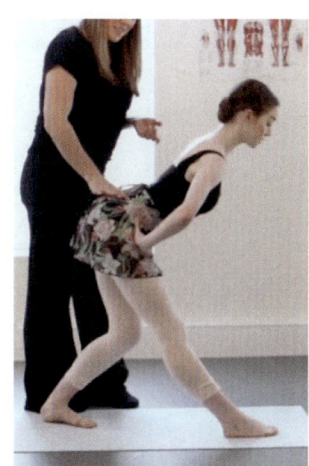 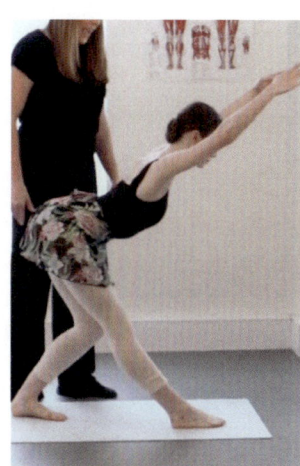

4. Turned Out with Thoracic Twist

- Starting in first position, add a twist and reach to the hamstring mobiliser.
- Step back onto your right foot, reaching your right hand across the front of the left foot.
- Focus on rotating the ribcage to add the thoracic spine into the mobilisation movement
- This addition can help you access a different part of the hamstrings that you won't get with the straight line mobilisers.
- If you start feeling tension down into the calf at any stage, just relax the foot flat to the floor.

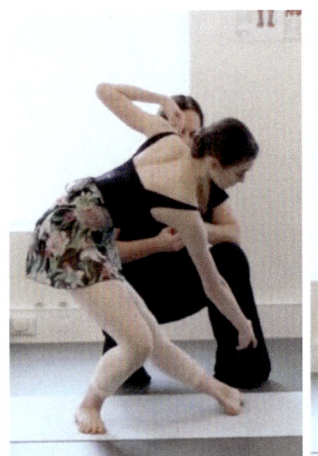
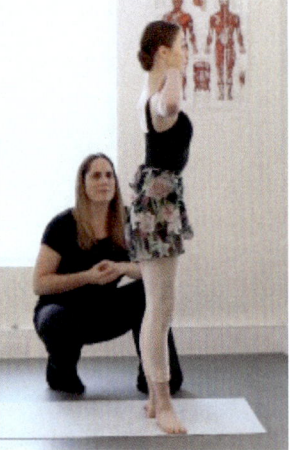
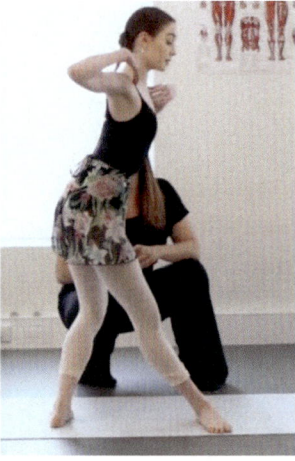
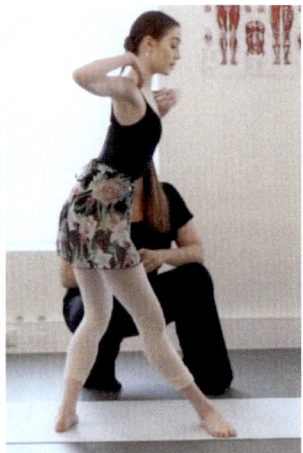

Notes:

_____
_____
_____
_____
_____
_____
_____
_____
_____
_____
_____
_____
_____
_____
_____

Isolate

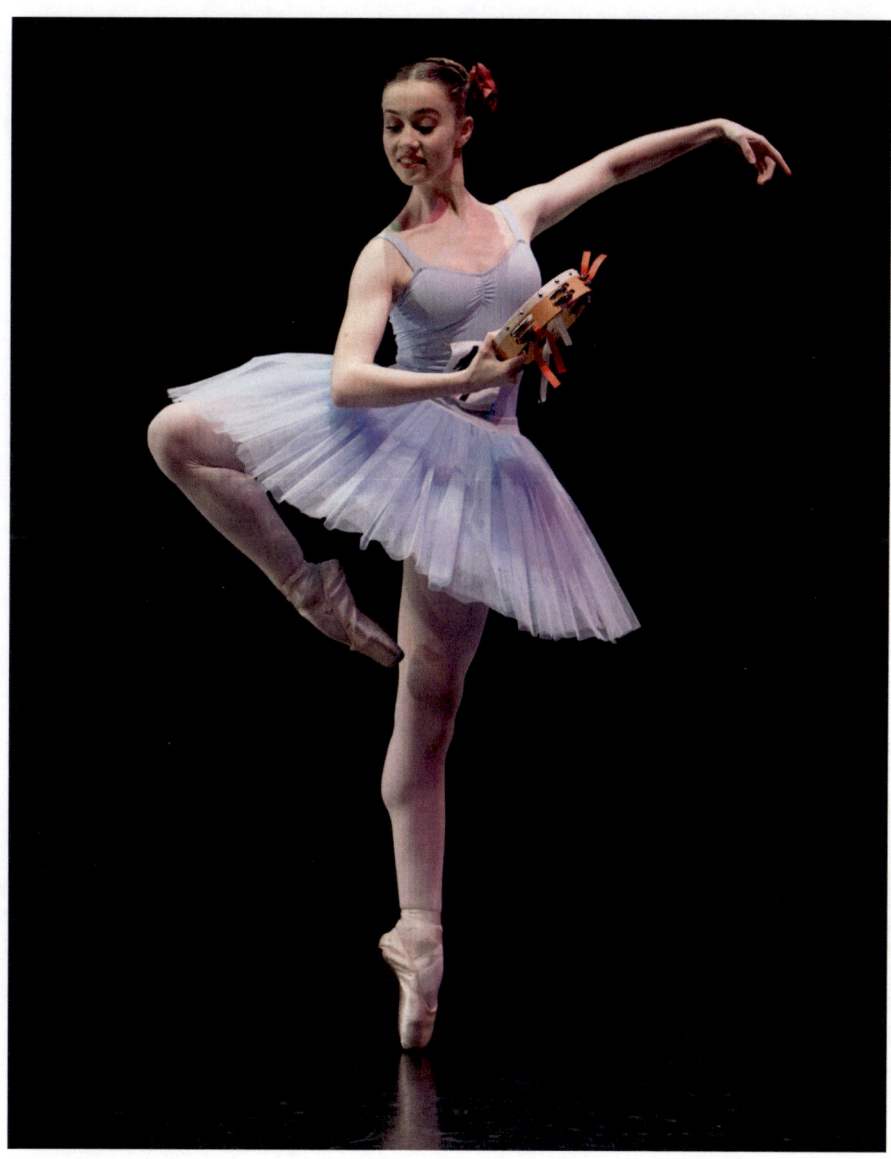

Isolating exercises are a very important part of this process. Correctly identifying any weaknesses in the deepest stabilising layers of the back, pelvis and hip can make an amazing difference in the quality of adage. Work on these isolation exercises for at least two weeks before moving on to the integration exercises, even if they feel easy. Please note all of the instructions about checking for over recruitment in other areas for each of these exercises. This is essential in finding the true isolation in each area which will give the effortless float to your extensions.

4 Point Sit Backs

This is a good test for the endurance and control in the deep back muscles, and is especially good for hyper-mobile individuals. Initially, this exercise may be done with a pole along the spine to get an awareness of maintaining neutral. Common mistakes include allowing the tail to tuck under, or sinking the upper back into extension, and the pole allows greater feedback to correct your placement in the early stages.

A lot of high level classical dancers tend to sit with the pelvis in a posterior tilt. Often we've been taught to scoop in through the front of the low abdomen and flatten out the low back. The problem with this is that it inhibits a lot of the important deep back stabilisers which in turn can lead to a lot of gripping in the front of the hips over time. Other dancers brace with the muscles in their upper back which limits mobility. This is really good exercise to see whether you tend to flatten your back or whether you tend to arch it too much.

- Start on your hands and knees, keeping your knees under your hips and your hands underneath your shoulders.
- Use a pole or broomstick to get awareness of where your back is, making sure you're in a neutral position.
- The pole should be in contact with the back of the rib cage and your sacrum. There will be a small gap between the low back and the pole, but make sure to keep the neck long and lengthened.
- Start the movement by folding in the hips, taking your sitting bones back to the wall behind you, keeping the spine in a neutral position.
- Try not to let the hips sink or the back flatten.
- If you tend to brace with the bigger back muscles, the ribcage will arch off the pole as you start moving the hips.
- If you lose control of the deep back muscles the low back will flatten when you start to flex the hips.
- Repeat about 10 times, checking the positioning of the spine in a mirror.
- Once you are confident with the control of your spine you may do this exercise without the pole.
- Try doing the exercise side on to the mirror or with a partner to check the positioning of your spine.

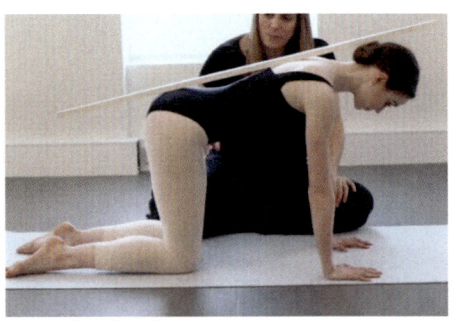
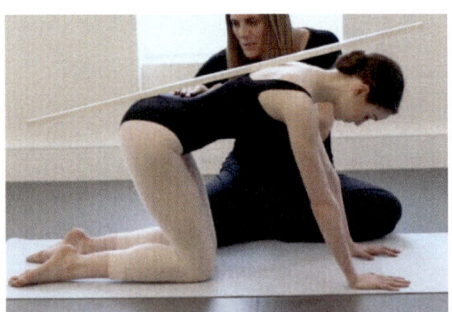
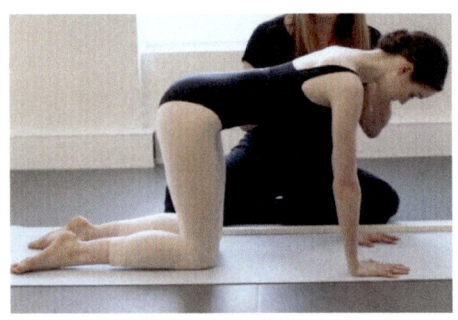

Cushion Squeezes

The Cushion Squeezes exercise will help isolate and strengthen your deep Adductor (Inner Thigh) muscles. A lot of dancers do not realise how important these muscles are when carrying their leg to the front. Finding subtle control of the deepest inner thigh muscles (Pectineus) will give you much more control and support when carrying the leg to the front, and will help take the weight away from the outside of the hip. This can help take the pressure off your TFL if they have been over working. Remember that optimal control of the hips requires a fine co-ordination of all of the muscles around the hips, rather than brute strength in any one group.

- Lie on your back, with feet hip width apart and in line with each other.
- Place one hand under your lower back, to feel if the big back muscles are turning on as you contract the inner things (this is very common).
- Place a small, soft, slightly deflated ball between your inner thighs, about halfway down the legs rather than between the knees.
- Maintaining gentle, natural breathing, focus on drawing your two thigh bones together to squeeze the ball.
- Use your fingertips to check that the big back muscles, TFL and gluteals stay relaxed.
- Hold for three slow breaths, allowing the low belly to rise and fall with each breath, before releasing the inner thigh contraction.
- Repeat 8 times, or until you start to fatigue. This usually occurs after just 3 or 4 repetitions when dancers first start with this exercise, as it really isolates the often under-used Pectineus.
- If the legs start to tremble, simply stop and rest for a few moments while you do one of the other exercises before trying again.
- Working on this exercise carefully will really improve your endurance and strength of the inner thighs.

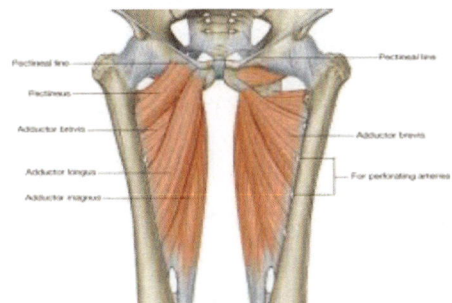

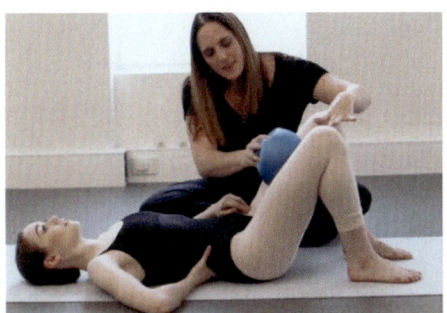

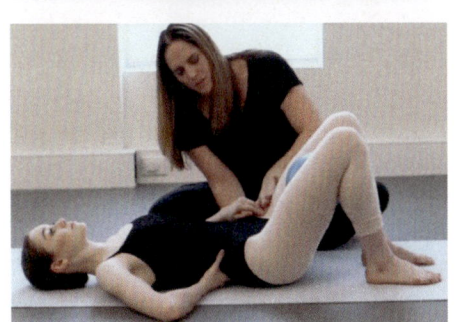

Note:
- Initially the ball must be placed quite low between your thighs, as it does tend to work its way up during this exercise.
- Monitor your TFL for over activity, especially if you have had issues with clicking in your hips.
- Neutral spine involves a gentle lift through the base of the spine, and a gentle drawing in and hollowing of the low pelvis, without flattening the back.
- While focussing on the inner thighs, make sure to keep the shoulders nicely open and relaxed.

QF Heel Squeeze

Often I ask dancers to show me where their turnout muscles are and I usually get a few interesting responses. Some dancers think that they are on top of the hamstrings, while others think they at the top of their bottom or the front of the hip. In reality your turnout muscles are really deep in the back of the hip. Knowing exactly where these are and how to activate them is really important when you are trying to learn how to control the leg en l'air.

Your Quadratus Femoris (QF) muscle is an important turnout muscle, that will help your standing/supporting leg and also helps control your turnout devant. This QF Heel Squeeze is an ideal exercise to become aware of and activate your QF muscle. It is ideally done before any other turnout exercises.

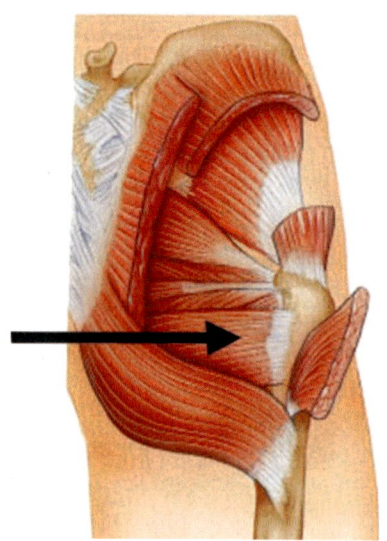

Your QF is also one of the most important muscles to find, train, and incorporate into technique following any hip injury. It helps stabilise the head of the femur back in the socket and is an essential deep turnout muscle when standing, working en fondu and for turnout en avant. There are many different ways to activate QF, but care must be taken to ensure that it is done with no pain and without any activation of other global stabilisers around the hip. Different individuals will have different coping strategies, so it is important to keep checking around the hip for hidden compensation strategies.

1. **Finding the QF**

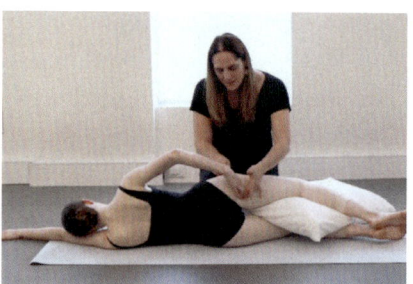

- Start on your side, with a cushion between your knees.
- Make sure that your thighbone is horizontal to the floor, supported by the cushion/pillow.
- Place your thumb on your greater trochanter, which is the highest knob of bone on the outside of the hip.
- Reach with your other fingers and place them on your sitting bone of that side of the pelvis.
- The QF muscle is halfway between these two points, in the gutter behind the greater trochanter.
- Use your fingers that were on the sitting bones to feel for your QF muscle deep in the back of the hip.
- You will need to use a decent amount of pressure to get through all of the superficial tissues.
- Make sure to try various different angles at the hip to find the one where your hip flexors and upper gluteals can be relaxed. This position is slightly different for everyone.

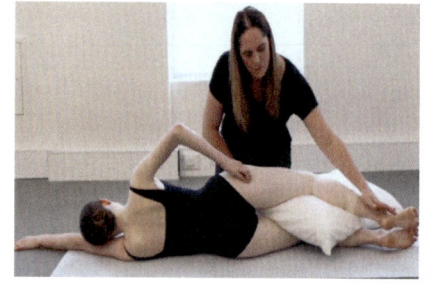

2. **Activating QF**

- To make sure the QF muscle is working effectively, ask your partner to lift your lower leg, internally rotating the thigh bone.
- Focussing on rotating the thigh bone in the socket, pull your foot down towards the floor against the resistance of your partners hand.
- Keep your fingers over the area of the QF muscle and see if you can feel a deep activation in the back of the hip.
- When activating correctly you should feel a slow, deep swelling of the muscle that builds up in intensity, rather than a sudden superficial gripping of the outer tissues.
- Repeat this movement a few times, making sure that the activation of the muscle is resulting in the actual movement of the leg, not just tightening the muscle.

3. **Performing the Exercise Yourself**

- Once you have found the correct activation, you can do a version of this exercise yourself.
- Stack your heels on top of each other, and use the previous cues to find the location of the QF
- Gently squeeze your heels together thinking of rotating the thigh bone in the socket.
- Keep your upper knee in contact with the cushion, rather than opening the legs.
- You should feel a deep thickening of the muscle under your fingertips.
- Hold for 3 breaths and then release, keeping your knees on the cushion throughout.
- Once you have the awareness to correctly activate the QF, use your fingers of your top hand to assess how much tone is being held in the front of your hips and the top of your gluteals. Both of these areas should be able to be kept relaxed when performing the subtle QF isolation exercise.

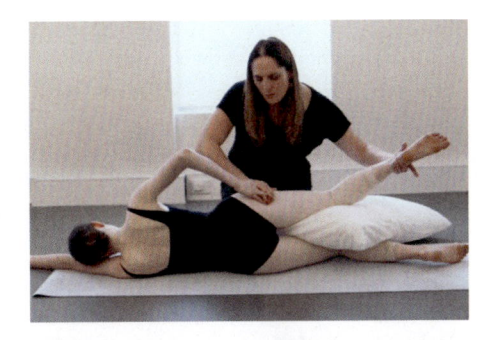

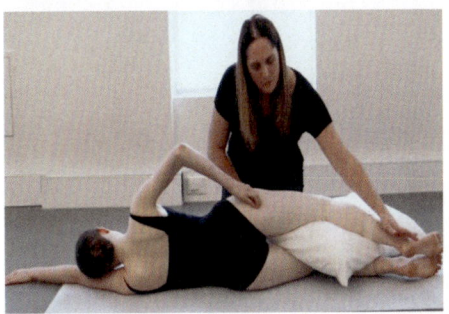

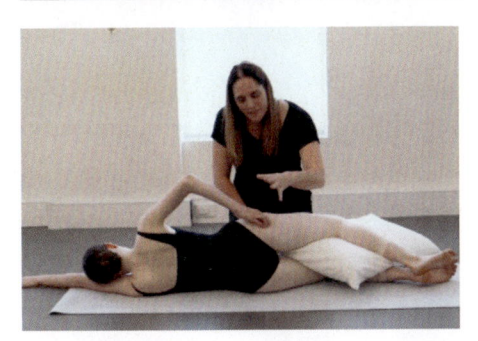

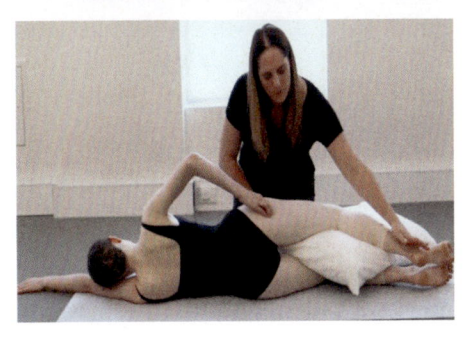

Note:
- Make sure Gluteus Medius and TFL remain soft throughout the exercise.
- If it is hard to keep them relaxed, try slightly altering the degree of flexion in the hips or repeating the trigger point release techniques and hip flexor mobilisers

Iliacus Suck - in Lying

The next exercise we are going to do is called the Iliacus Suck. A lot of people have never even heard of their Iliacus muscle, but it is very important in controlling your extensions. It's not really something that people talk about when they're in ballet class, but knowing a bit more about the detailed anatomy of your hip flexors can really help integrating their action into your adage.

One of my old teachers used to say to "lift from your abs" when your lifting the leg to the front. I used to think that this was impossible as your abdominals don't attach down onto your leg. What I think she was trying to explain is to get a sensation of scooping and connection deep in the abdomen, however unfortunately she just didn't explain that in a way that made sense to my 14 year old brain. To make it easier to understand and conceptualise, I'm going to explain the actual anatomy and that will help you find the feeling that we're looking for in this exercise.

If you look at a model of a pelvis, your Psoas Major attaches onto the front of the Lumbar Spine and then comes forward to the front of the hip. Your Iliacus starts from inside the bowl of the pelvis before coming forward to to join with the tendon of the Psoas Major, creating your Iliopsoas tendon. This tendon attaches onto the inner aspect of your upper thigh bone, making it instrumental in flexing the hip.

These two muscles (Psoas Major and Iliacus) are what I have found to be the secret to beautiful high lifted extensions. To achieve that floating sensation we are going to use the Iliacus to help stabilise the hip back into the socket and then use the Psoas Major to help fold the hip. Some dancers manage to achieve the subtle coordination of them naturally, however most others need to specifically train them.

First we will practise the Iliac Suck in lying, and then in standing, before transferring it through to your développé devant later.

Assisted Version:

Initially it helps to work with a partner to get the direction of activation correct. Once you have this, you may work on the exercise alone.
- Start in lying, with one foot on the floor, and the other leg bent to 90 degrees with the foot on a chair.
- The partner will use both hands to gently traction the thigh bone up towards the ceiling.
- The dancer will oppose this traction drawing the thighbone back down and feel the hip heavy in the socket.

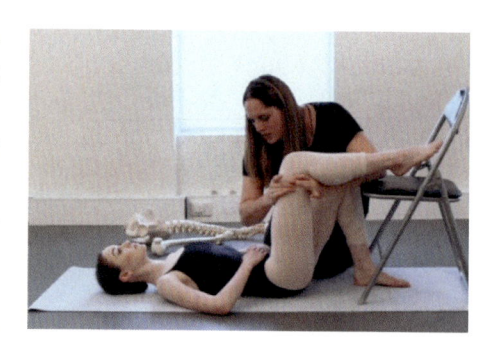

Independent Version

- Lie on your back, with one foot on a chair or Swiss ball, making sure the thigh bone is vertical.
- Keep the spine in neutral, with a very gentle lift in the low back to ensure activation of the deep back stabilisers.
- Using your hand, feel the outside of your TFL and top of the thigh, making sure all of those muscles stay soft.
- Visualise the thighbone being very heavy, and feel it slide back deep in the socket
- Repeat this movement a few times to become familiar with it. The movement is very subtle, with just a few mm in actual movement.
- When performing the exercise correctly, you will feel a gentle thickening inside the hip bone of the working leg, while all the surrounding muscles stay relaxed
- Once awareness of the hip suck is achieved add in a gentle knee float.
- Perform the hip suck, then allow the hip to flex, folding deep in the socket.
- The movement should be effortless and be controlled by the deepest hip flexors (Iliacus and Psoas Major) rather than by using the muscles on the outside of the hip.
- Do not worry too much about keeping the thigh in perfect parallel if the is any compression in the front of the hip.
- If your hips are very externally rotated it is ok to let the knee drift out slightly during the hip fold. Due to variations in anatomy the thigh bone will float up in a slightly turned up position.
- Repeat 8 times on each side, constantly checking for excessive gripping around the hip as the deepest muscles start to fatigue.

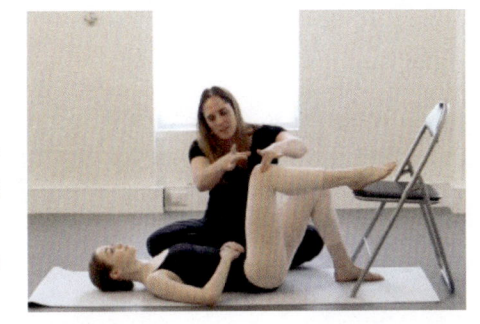

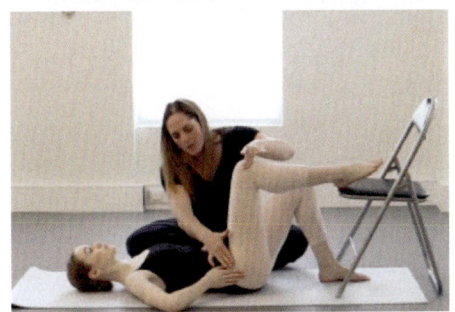

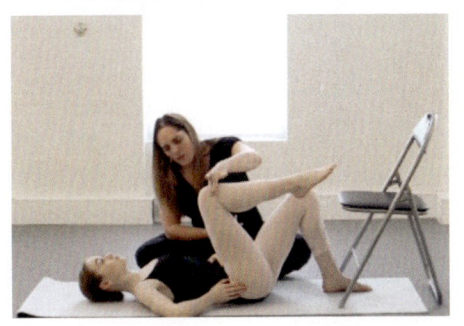

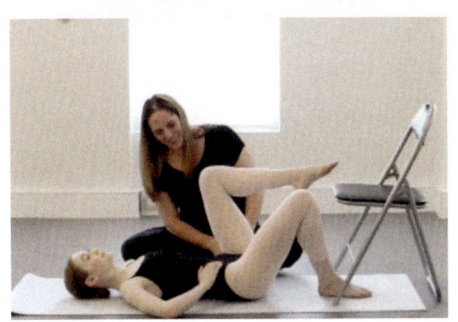

Note:
- Breathing must be natural and not forced
- Make sure you stay a little lifted under the lumbar spine throughout.
- Use hands to monitor over activity of the global back muscles (Erector Spine) and the superficial hip muscles (TFL, Gluteals)
- When the knee float is added in, make sure not to flex the spine or grip with the front of the hip.

Psoas Activation in 4 Point

This next exercise used to be involved in one of our turnout programs, but I rarely give it to dancers these days. I included it here to explain why I don't do it so much anymore and if you are doing it some points to be careful of. Once you know how to do it properly, you'll understand where the benefit can be but also the risks if you do it poorly. It's basically a hands and knees version of the Iliacus suck and float.

1. **Basic Activation**

- Start on hands and knees, keeping the spine in a neutral position, taking care not to hyper-extend the elbows.
- Accept your weight slightly onto your left leg, then draw the right thigh bone back into the socket with the same subtle sucking feeling as in the previous exercise
- Once you can master this, and the right knee clears the floor, float the right knee forward.
- Make sure to keep the pelvis stable and still. Avoid hitching the hip of the working leg, or flattening the lumbar spine.
- If this is happening, this is going to actually build up all the muscles that we don't want to use rather than the ones we're trying to find.
- Get your partner to check that the outer hip muscles, and especially the TFL are relaxed. Flexion must come from the deepest hip flexors to make this exercise effective.

2. **With Resistance**

- This exercise can be progressed by the addition of a resistance band around the knee, however this should only be done if the outer hip remains relaxed.
- A lot of students will flatten the back and hitch the hip when drawing the knee forward. This can create a lot of tension around the outside of the hip, which is what we are trying to avoid in all our isolation exercises.
- Whilst doing this exercise, please make sure that you're thinking of all of these things and that you're not actually doing something that could be detrimental.

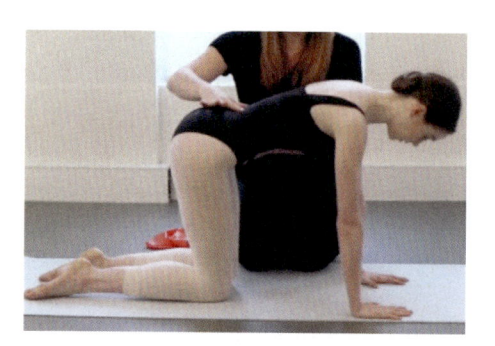

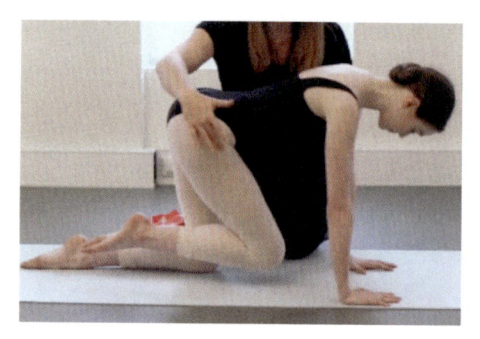

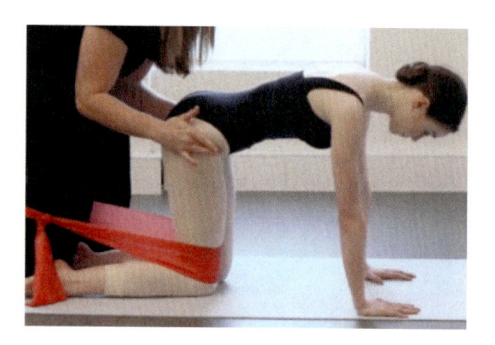

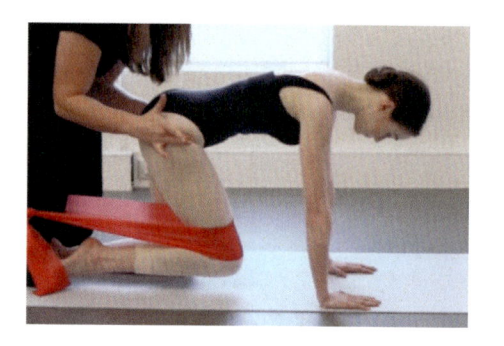

Turnout with Foot on the Wall

The last exercise in the isolation sequence is all about tying the previous isolation exercises together. This exercise is a good way to really learn how each muscle we have been working on actually supports your leg in a développé devant, because in the beginning they can seem a little abstract. You will need at least 90 degrees of hamstring flexibility to do this exercise comfortably. If this is difficult for you initially, focus more on the mobilisation exercises until your range improves.

1. Basic Rotation

- Lie close to the wall, with one leg up the wall and your finger tips on your hip bone.
- With the most minimal amount of effort, think of rotating the elevated leg in the socket, feeling the deep turnout muscles wrapping around underneath.
- Aim for the least amount of effort to get the leg to rotate, rather than gripping with all of the muscles.
- Relax the leg and let it return to parallel.
- Repeat this a few times, to get used to the feeling of the thighbone rotating easily in the socket.

2. Adding the Iliac Hip Suck and Float

- Rotate the leg using your deep rotators and centre the hip in the socket with the Iliacus Hip Suck.
- Maintaining neutral spine, and with the big back muscles relaxed, float the foot off the wall by gently engaging your Psoas Major.
- Maintain regular breathing, and again focus on the most subtle control of the leg, with no extra activation around the hip.
- Lower it down and release to parallel.

3. Adding the Foot

- Once you are confident in the activation and control around the hip, you can add on the pointe through demi pointe exercise, while the leg is floating, articulating slowly through the foot.
- This is a much more challenging variation, so make sure to keep monitoring the activity of the superficial muscles around the hip.

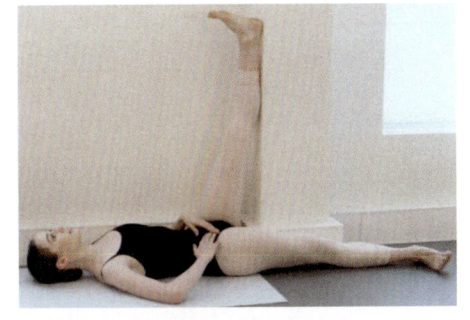

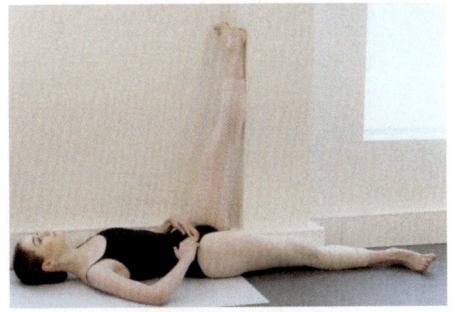

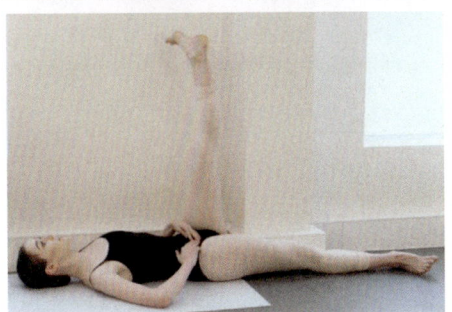

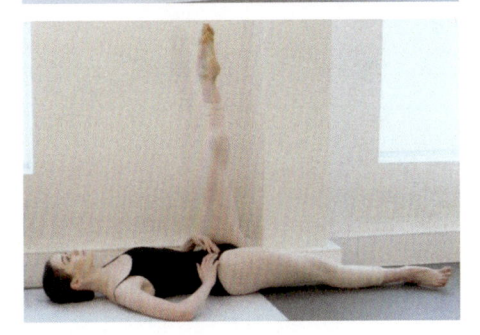

Notes:

Integrate

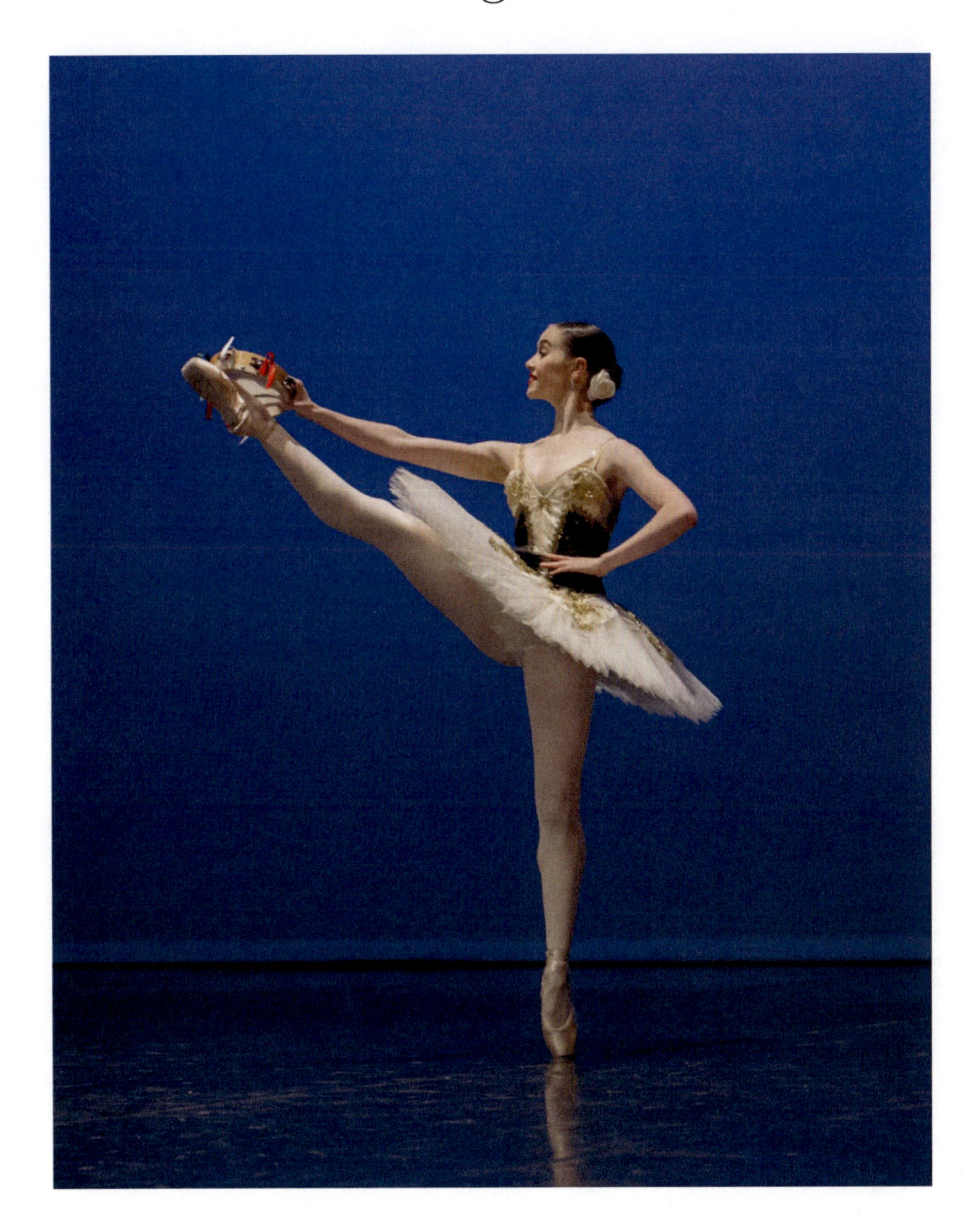

The Integration stage is where you start tying things together. This stage is all about developing new muscle patterning to override your old habits and motor programs to transform your dancing. Each exercise is carefully chosen to incorporate elements of the previous isolation exercises and start working deeper into range. Please keep in mind throughout this section that none of these exercises should cause any pain or discomfort.

Waiter Bow

This 'Waiter Bow' exercise takes the movement that we were doing with the '4 Point Sit Back' and brings it into standing. One of the biggest issues I see in dancers is the tendency to tuck the pelvis too much in order to try and get the leg higher. When you do a full développé devant you will add a slight tuck of the pelvis, however if you are tucking to get to 90 degrees or just a little bit higher, you'll never get much higher than that. The higher you can get the leg without a tuck, the better, and then when you add on a subtle tuck you can take the leg to full height. Basically, the further forward you can go with this exercise, maintaining a neutral spine, the higher you will be able to get your leg without tucking.

- Start standing in parallel, with neutral spine with the knees soft.
- Get your partner to place the pole against your spine. You want to think of the tail bone and the ribcage touching the pole, with a little bit of a gap at the area of the low back.
- Soften your knees maintaining neutral spine.
- Watching your spinal profile in the mirror, and hinge forward from your hips, letting the heads of the thigh bones sink back in the sockets and fold in the front of the hips.
- Make sure to keep the spine in neutral but take care not to over grip with the low back.
- If the Multifidus is weak, you will tend to flatten the low back when hinging forward.
- If you are bracing with the big back muscles (Erector Spinae) the upper back will arch away from the pole.
- Only lean forward as far as you can control the back in neutral.
- Return to standing, and repeat 10 times.

Variations:
1. Perform the exercise with just a minimal forward lean, with soft knees in parallel
2. Aim to get the spine horizontal to the floor with the knees slightly bent
3. Aim to get the spine horizontal to the floor with the knees straight (not hyperextended)
4. Aim for full range with spine in neutral and knees straight
5. Try in parallel, turned out and turned in.

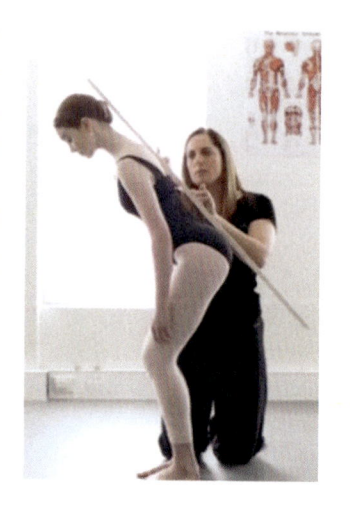

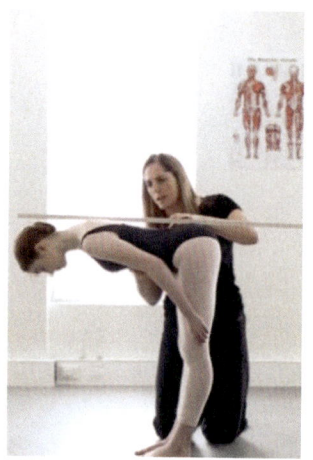

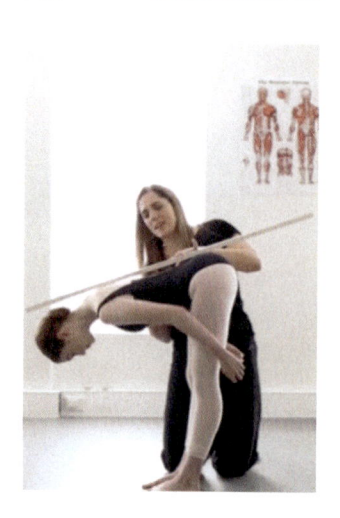

Cushion Squeezes with Leg Extension and Rotation

This next exercise adds in extension and rotation of the leg to the original Cushion Squeeze exercise. In all of these exercises we focus on deep, subtle coordination around the hips rather than building brute strength. You don't want to build up too much bulk around the hips, but instead want to feel a deep, subtle connection in the hips to help support your extensions to the front.

- Start lying on your back, with the ball between your inner thighs.
- Slowly squeeze the ball, imagining the thigh bones coming together in parallel.
- Check that the front of the hips are relaxed and maintain regular breathing.
- Maintaining the inner thigh activation, slowly straighten out the right knee.
- Note that the hip flexors of the working leg will activate, but the supporting hip should stay relaxed.
- Rotate your working leg in the socket, really feeling the connection from your inner thighs to your turnout muscles.
- Maintaining the inner thigh activation, bring the leg back into parallel.
- Slowly bend the knee to bring the foot back down to the floor and then release the inner thigh contraction.
- To check you're doing this exercise correctly, you can place your hands on your hip bones to check for twisting of the pelvis, or use your fingers to assess for overactivity of the hip flexors or global back muscles.

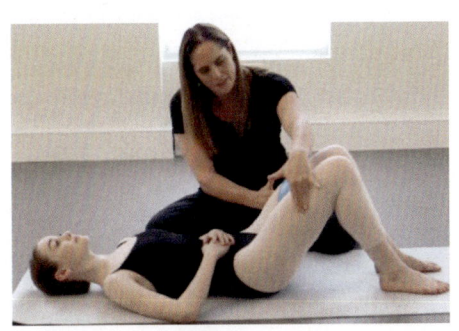

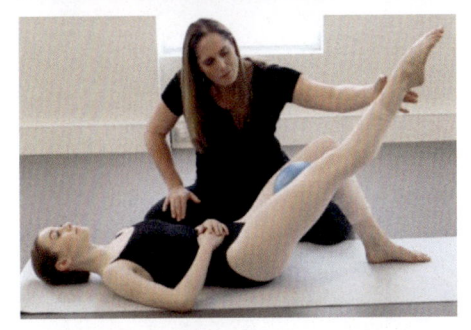

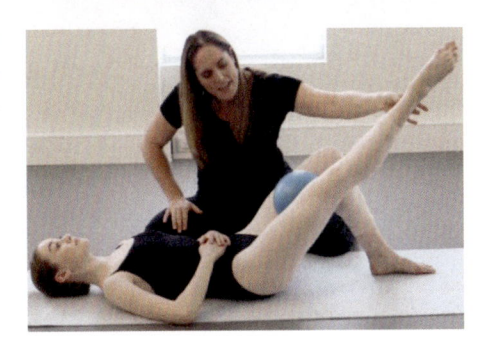

4 Point Turnout with Endurance

This exercise is designed to build endurance for maintaining turnout to the front, and is also an excellent exercise for your arabesque.

- Start on your hands and knees, in neutral with the knees directly under the hips. Keep a little arch down through the lower back, broad across the shoulders, while remaining open through the front of the chest. Stay long through the neck, elbows slightly soft (not hyper extended)
- Slowly extend your leg out the back and place the foot on demi pointe,
- Then rotate the supporting leg around, wrapping the deep turnout muscles.

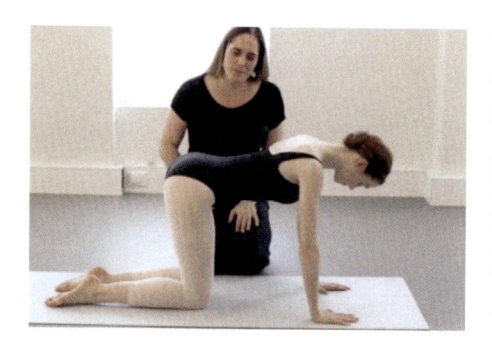

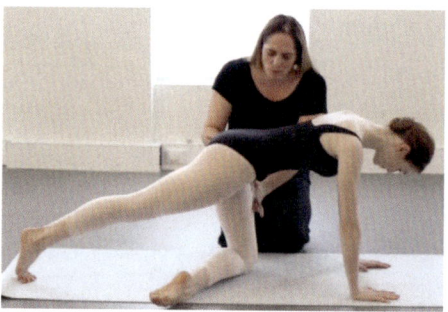

- Transfer your weight onto your supporting leg and float the working leg up in parallel.
- Flex the foot and rotate the thigh bone in the socket, keeping the hips square.
- Point through demi-point and then lower the leg slowly in turnout.
- Replace the foot to the floor, come back to a 4 point position, and then rest back in child's pose.

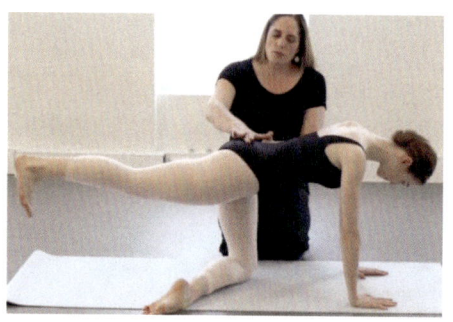

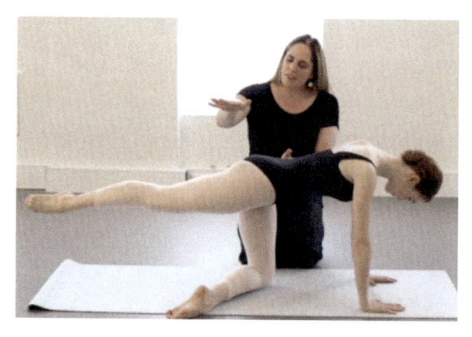

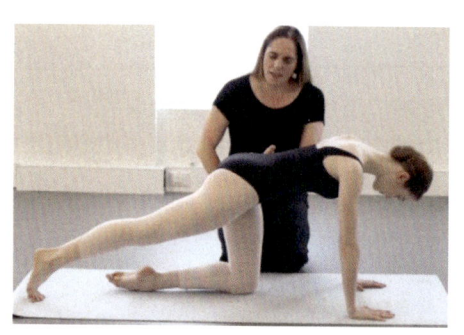

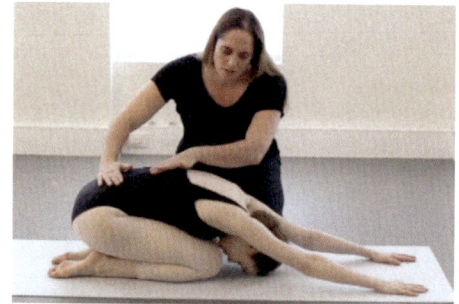

Cushion Squeezes with Oblique Curl

This exercise is really important for activating your Anterior Oblique System (AOS) which is an important dynamic connection between your inner thighs and your opposite oblique abdominals. An effective AOS can really help you control your extensions to the front.

- Start lying on your back, with the spine in neutral
- Place your feet hip width apart and your hands behind your head, elbows wide.
- Place the ball between your thighs and do a gentle cushion squeeze, keeping slightly lifted through the low back and connected through the front.
- Keeping one elbow on the ground, and both elbows wide, gently curl the ribcage up and across bringing the left ribcage toward the right hip/inner thigh.
- Focus on feeling a connection from the oblique abdominals of one side through to the inner thighs of the opposite side.
- Exhale through the movement to help connect to your deep abdominals and pelvic floor
- Make sure to keep the low abdomen slightly hollowed, not bulging as you curl up.
- If it is difficult to keep the low abdomen gently drawing in, or just to check your form, place the hand of the lifted shoulder down on your low tummy to help improve your awareness.
- Release, switch hands and repeat to the other side.
- Repeat at least 8 times to each side.
- Once you have good activation and are confident that the low abdomen is not bulging, try reaching your free hand across to the outside of your opposite leg.
- Keep a gentle sensation of subtly activating the deep low back muscles throughout this exercise, rather than flattening the back into the floor.

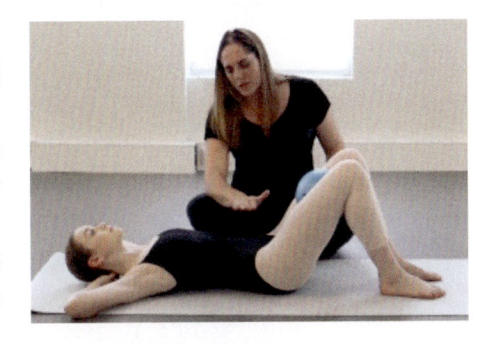

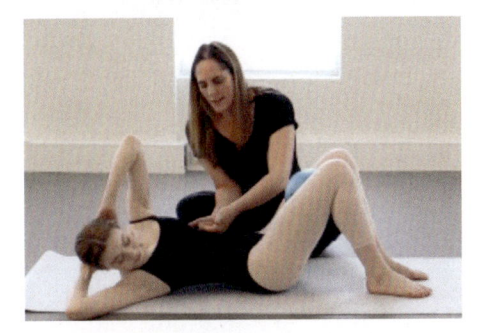

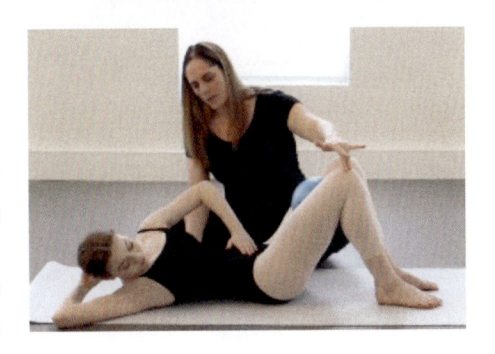

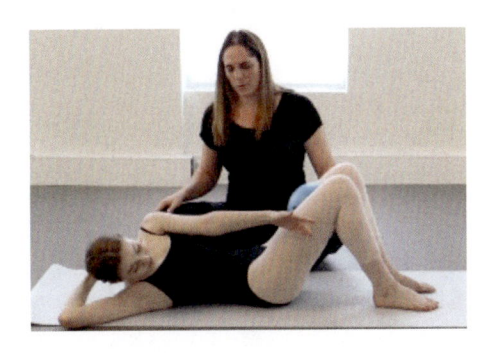

Standing Iliacus Suck

Before going into the Standing Iliac Suck it is a good idea to go through the lying version. Just do a couple on each side to reactivate the Iliacus before trying to recruit it in standing. Remember that Iliacus works subtly to draw the thigh bone back into the hip socket to give you more control of the leg en l'air and help offload the superficial hip flexors.

Lying Version:
- Lying on your back, with one foot on a chair, making sure the thigh bone is vertical.
- Use your fingertips to feel the outside of your hip and top of the thigh to ensure these areas stay soft and relaxed.
- Visualise the thigh bone sinking deep into the socket and then gently float the knee towards you, keeping the spine in neutral and the TFL relaxed.
- Slowly release and place the foot back on the chair.

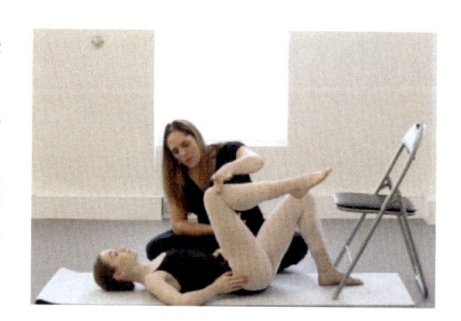

Standing Version:
- To perform this in standing, stand on the left leg and place the right foot onto demi-pointe. Stay lifted through the centre and lengthened through the sides of the waist.
- Connect the right hip bone deep into the socket with the Iliacus suck, then float the thigh bone up towards 90 degrees, maintaining natural breathing.
- Make sure to keep lifted through the tiny deep low back muscles, maintaining the spine in neutral.
- Make sure not to tuck the pelvis to lift the thigh bone. This will destabilise the lower back and put a lot of load into the front of the hip.
- Do not worry if the lifted leg does not stay completely in parallel. With some anatomical variations it will deviate slightly into external rotation.
- Repeat on alternate legs, approximately 4-8 on each side depending on your current strength and endurance.

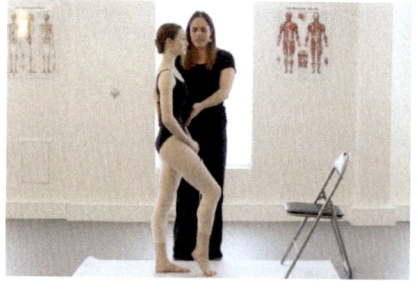

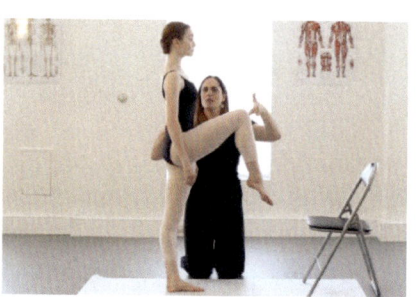

Note:
- As you get stronger you will be able to take the thigh bone past 90 degrees. The higher you can take the thigh bone with the spine in neutral. the more effortless your développé devant will become!
- You are aiming for the most effortless movement you can make, using as little muscle as possible to get a sensation of the thigh bone floating up. This is the feeling we want to get when we start doing our extensions devant later on in the program.

Adult Crawling Sequence

"Adult Crawling" is a great exercise to help develop connections in the Anterior Oblique and Posterior Oblique slings which normally get developed when babies learn to crawl. If a baby misses out a significant period of crawling for any reason, this may affect their natural deep core stability later on in life. Even if a baby does have a good period of crawling, it is important that we continue to strengthen the cross patterns later on in life.

Technically 'Adult Crawling' is not the same as regular 4 point crawling but it's a great variation to take the load out of your knees. This is especially important for adolescent dancers between the age of about 11 to 14 as knee issues are common when you do lots of growing. This is also good for some adults who do not like being on their knees too much due to degenerative changes. This exercise develops the cross patterning through the front (Anterior Oblique System) and back (Posterior Oblique System) to develop the control needed to control your adage.

The series includes six different variations. Try working through them, but stop at the one that you can do quite well. It is better to be practicing a good movement pattern, than be struggling too hard. Once you can achieve one version well you can gradually move through the full sequence.

Level 1 - Basic:
- Stand on your right leg, and float the left knee up to have the thigh horizontal.
- Keeping the hips and shoulders square, press the right hand into the inside of the left leg. Press quite firmly so you can feel your inner thighs and your obliques (Anterior Oblique System) connect.
- Hold for 3 seconds. Keep lifted through the low back so that it stays in neutral and maintain natural breathing.
- Place the left foot down just in front of the right big toe and then repeat on the other side.
- Note that the arch of the supporting foot will tend to activate automatically. This is really helpful in hypermobile people who struggle to find good dynamic arch control.

Level 2 - With Rotation:
- Repeat as for Level 1 but add in a rotation of the chest toward the lifted leg while keeping the hips square.
- The head can stay either facing forward, or rotate to the side.
- Keep the lumbar spine in neutral, and make sure not to extend the thoracic spine.
- Repeat 8 times on each side, pressing firmly to activate your AOS.

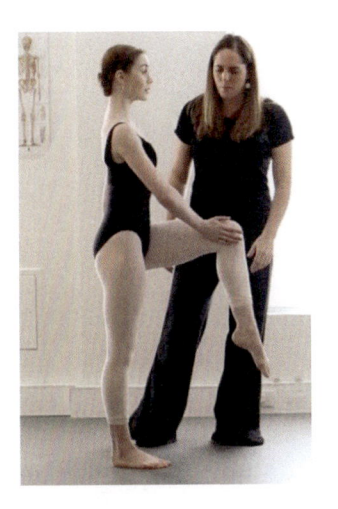

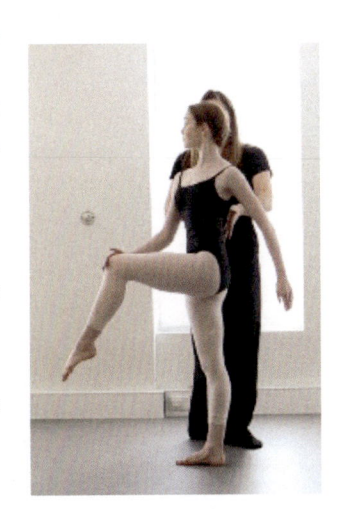

Level 3 - With Toe Tap:
- Start with a knee float and rotation as for Level 2.
- Place the hands on the hips and go into a little fondu extending the lifted leg behind you, tapping the toe to the floor.
- When you tilt forward, think of floating through the back of the rib cage a tiny bit, getting the same feeling as you did with the 'Waiter Bow' exercise.
- Try to keep everything nice and square. Keep centred through the pelvis, lengthened through the side waist, low back in neutral and relaxed through the back of the ribcage.
- Bring the working leg back up into the initial position of knee float and rotation, and then change legs.

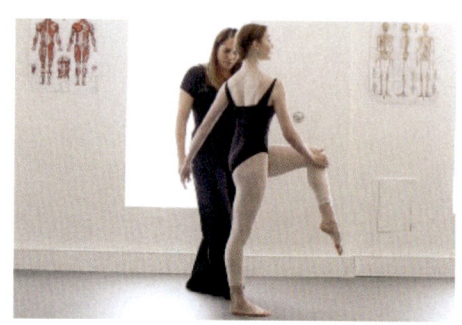

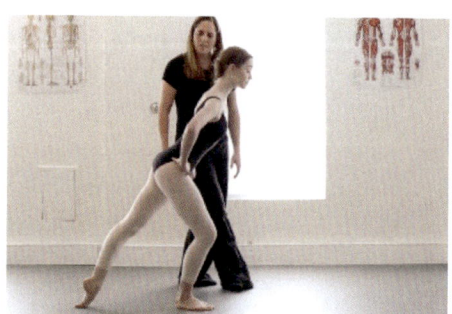

Level 4 - The Pedestrian Version:
- In the 'pedestrian' version the foot is flexed and the legs are in parallel.
- Lift the left leg, bringing the right arm forward and taking the left one arm back, elbow high, rotating the chest towards the lifted leg.
- Reverse the arms, taking the working leg behind you, still flexed and in parallel, rotating the rib cage towards the supporting leg.
- Come back up, repeating the first position, then replace the foot to the floor and repeat to the other side.
- Making sure you're staying nice and centred and allowing a beautiful spiral rotation throughout the movement.
- This version will activate your Anterior Oblique System to the front, and your Posterior Oblique System (Lattissimus Dorsi and the opposite Gluteus Maximus), to the back.
- This version really starts to develop coordination of the deep collective centre, with a dynamically stabled spine over top.
- Make sure to keep your back leg in parallel. If you're classically trained it may feel strange, however this will actually target the deep rotators of your supporting leg more.

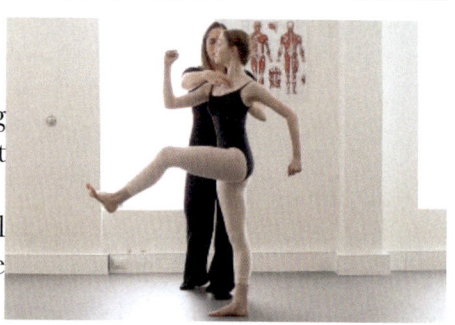

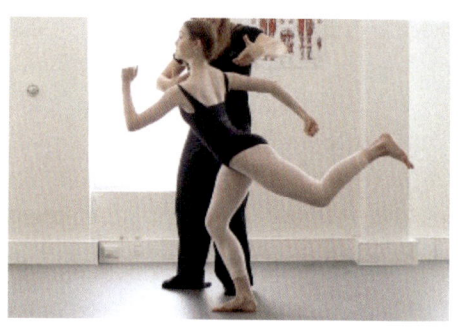

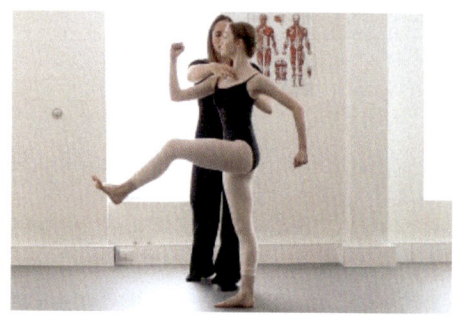

Level 5 - Horizontal T:
- Start as you did for Level 4, but as you pass the leg to the back extend it into a horizontal T with the spine in neutral.
- Try and keep the hips nice and square, the back leg in parallel, and avoid extending the upper back.
- Bring the working leg back the the front and then replace to the floor.
- Repeat 8 times on other side.
- Don't worry if you have a few little wobbles when working on this variation, that's actually part of finding your centre.
- This version really helps develop dynamic stability on that supporting side, as well as solidifying through those cross patterns.

Level 6 - Aeroplane:
- Begin as for Level 5, all the way until the horizontal T shape.
- Slowly rotate your upper body towards the supporting leg keeping the arms extended.
- Make sure to rotate the chest, not just swing the arms and keep the hips square as the upper body is rotating.
- Rotate the chest towards the lifted leg, then back towards the supporting leg before recovering back to the starting position with the knee lifted to the front
- Keep neutral in the lower back and deep connection in the front of the supporting hip.
- This version teaches the spine to be able to move whilst being stable, rather than bracing for control, which results in a rigid locked off centre.
- Any wobbles simply indicate that you haven't been doing exercises focused on this dynamic control with the spine. Play with a couple of those variation, see which one you find most comfortable and just work on gradually improving through the series.

Note:
- Try to maintain natural breathing throughout
- Move slowly and deliberately in and out of each position
- You should be able to do each stage comfortably for the full length of the room, heel to toe, before progressing onto the next version.

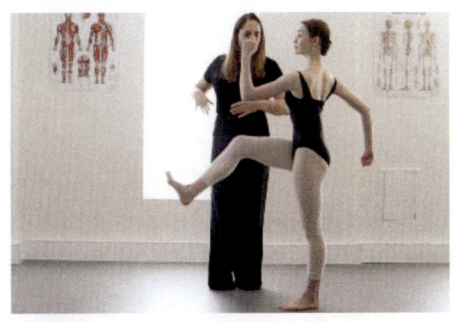

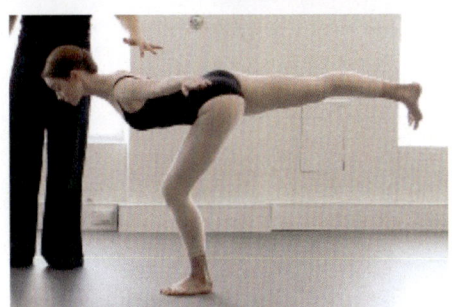

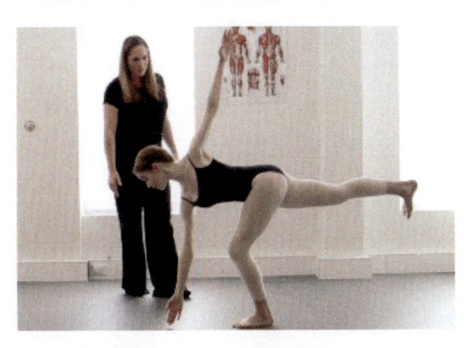

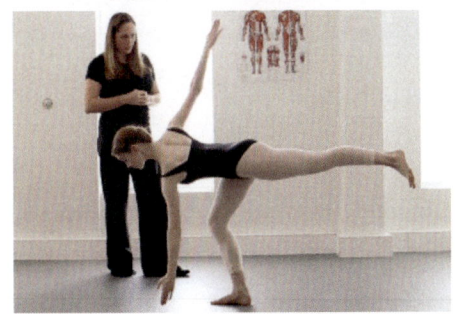

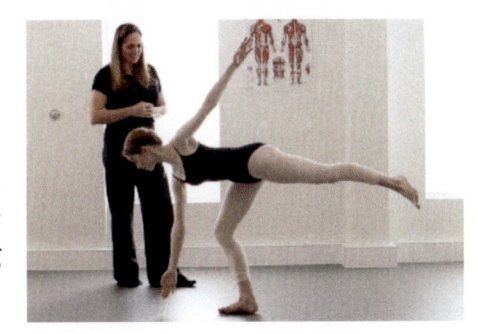

Notes:

Function

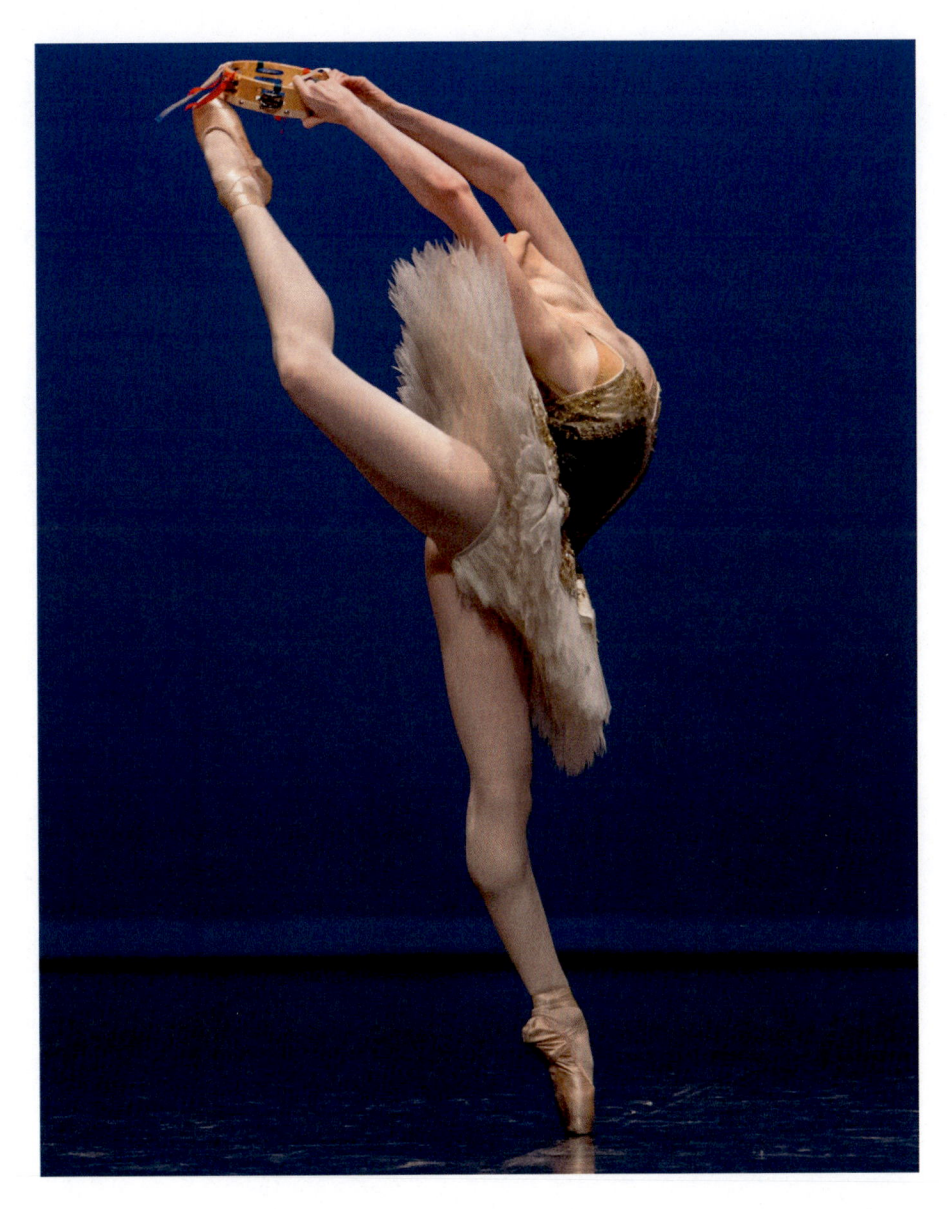

In the Functional section we take all of the elements that you have been working on and bring them all together to develop the patterns of movement needed to give you an effortless nature to your adage. Once the correct mobilisation of the area is achieved, you have isolated each necessary muscle group, and integrated them into the patterns needed, the functional exercises should be a whole lot easier. Our aim it to get past the conscious activation of all of the previous exercises, and become "unconsciously competent" in all of the elements, to allow you to have seamless technique, while focusing on your artistry and the story that is being told. After all, isn't that the whole point of dance?

QF Transfer with Port De Bras

Once you have mastered this exercise, it is really nice to do when you are warming up in the morning before class, to help activate and wake up your deep stabilisers in a functional way before you start going into class. It helps develop functional activation of your QF without over gripping other muscles around the hips. Adding on a beautiful Port De Bras to this exercise really highlights whether you are gripping on with outer abdominals or if you have found the connection to your true core. For this exercise I like using a big Swiss ball. If you don't have one of these you can use a smaller ball, simply place it behind your sacrum and keep the upper back off the wall.

Basic Version:
- Place a large Swiss ball, or small stability ball on the wall behind you just above your sacrum.
- Keep the spine in neutral and bend both your knees.
- Focusing on the deep rotators of the supporting leg, slowly transfer your weight onto one foot.
- Think of collecting the centre, lifting slightly through the low back to maintain neutral, and adding the Iliacus Suck to float the working leg to 90 degrees.
- Slowly lower the foot back down to the floor and then transfer to the other side.

Advanced Version:
- This variation adds in some upper body with a port de bra. This helps to ensure that you are not gripping with your outer abdominals for stability
- Plié in parallel, keeping lifted through the low back, and transfer onto one leg as for the previous version.
- Float your arms up through first position and then up to fifth, extending the upper back a little over the ball in a small cambré.
- Try adding a gentle Port De Bras including a small side bend over to each side.
- This one is really challenging because you need to make subtle adjustments as the centre of gravity changes.

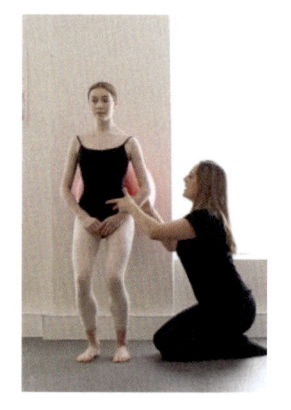

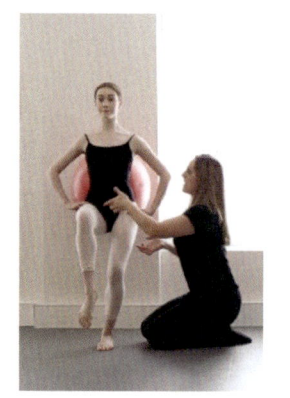

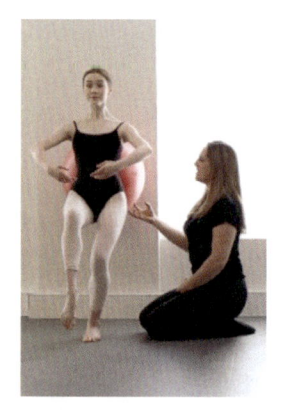

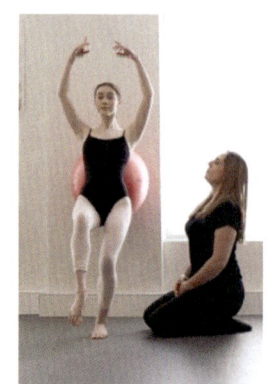

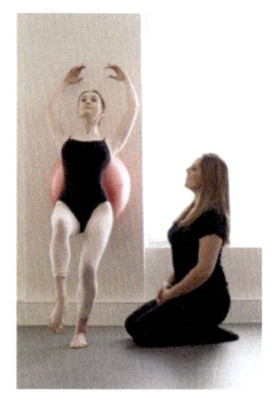

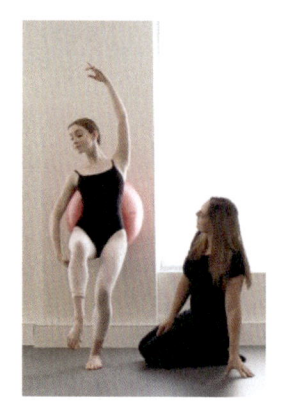

Développé Devant in Lying

This exercise is very good way to refine your technique and correct any 'cheating' habits that you may have used in the past in an attempt to get your leg higher. Performing this exercise on the ground allows you to create a new movement pattern which is much more focused on centralising the hip, finding your deep rotators and flexing the hip using your Psoas Major. Combining these elements in sequence, but in a more abstract position, helps create a new motor pattern in your brain, rather than modifying your old one, which helps retrain your patterning for performing développé much faster. As there is less effect of gravity on the working leg, you can learn how to subtly coordinate the correct muscles around the hip to place the leg in a good position, so that when you return to standing, it is much easier..

Make sure you are nice and mobile through your hamstrings, and have woken up all of the deep core and hip muscles before attempting this. This is a really good exercise for those dancers who have lots of mobility but who struggle to control their leg at the front. It helps gather all the things we've been talking about in sequence so that you can transfer them directly into your dancing.

Level 1:

- Start lying on the ground, with feet in fifth position.
- Flex your supporting leg and keep the back border of the foot engaged with the ground, so that your standing leg turnout muscles are working.
- If you do not have the available range to have the foot flat to the floor, simply visualise this, and make sure to keep the deep rotators engaged throughout.
- Slowly peel the right leg up into a retiré focussing on keeping flat through the hips.
- Make sure to use all available range through this movement, rather than lifting the leg in a turned in position and dropping it out in the retiré position.
- Slowly, unfold the leg to a développé devant at 90 degrees, making sure that the hips stay nice and square.
- Rotate your leg into parallel and then back into turnout three times.
- Make sure to keep connected to your centre and use your deep hip rotators to isolate the leg in the socket.
- Slowly lower the leg in turnout, then repeat on the other side.
- You only need to do 1-2 repetitions of each variation.

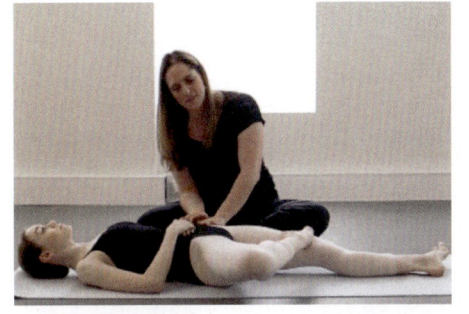

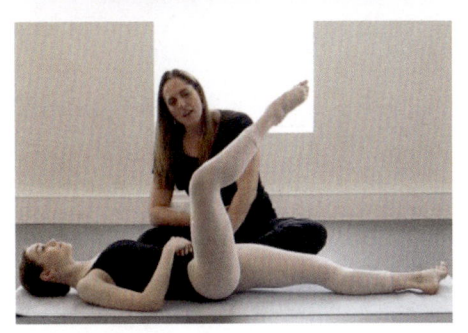

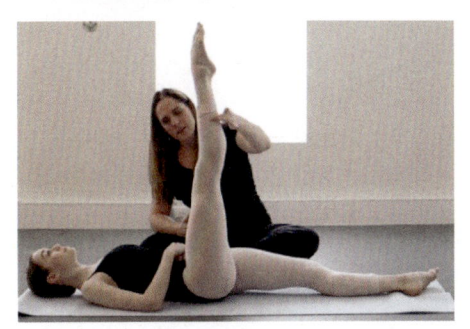

Level 2:

- Start as for Level 1, peeling up through retiré to a développé devant at 90 degrees.
- Using your opposite hand, mount your lifted leg to where you'd like your développé to be.
- Take special note of your placement, keeping the thigh bone really rotated into the socket.
- Make sure you don't hitch the hip of the working leg up.
- Think of keeping a little lift through the low back to activate those deep muscles.
- Maintain a deep connection with your psoas from the front of the hip through to the front of the spine.
- Once you have found the correct position, slowly let go of your leg and see if you can maintain the position of the leg with your Psoas and Iliac connection.
- Lengthen the back of the knee, keeping the whole leg nicely rotated and foot fully pointed.
- Hold for a breath or two, then lower the leg to the floor.

Level 3:

- Start as for Level 1, but as you unfold from the retiré, place your leg where you'd like it to be when standing.
- This will require a deeper engagement of Iliac and Psoas Major to place the thigh bone above 90 degrees.
- Maintain the deep rotation in the socket, deep connection in the front of the hip, and unfold the leg keeping it in midline.
- Lengthen the back of the knee of the supporting leg and ensure turnout is maintained.
- Pause for a few breaths, before lowering the leg.

This exercise is more of a neural activation process than a loaded muscle exercise. It's more about learning how use your brain to connect to the required muscles rather than doing repetitions under load to create strength. When training the hip it's more about subtle coordination of all of the muscles around the hip rather than brute strength. There should never be any pain following any of these exercises but you will feel a lot more woken up around the hips and should feel more stable when you come to standing

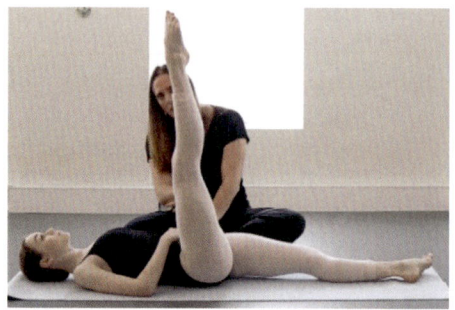

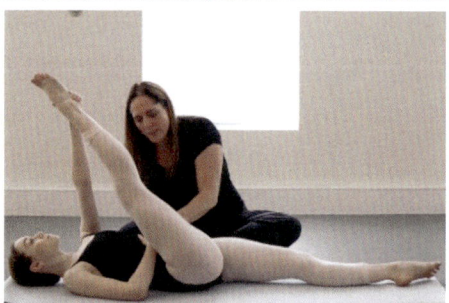

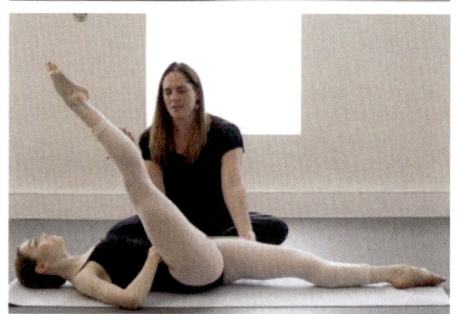

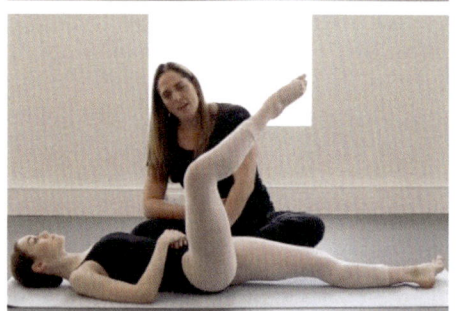

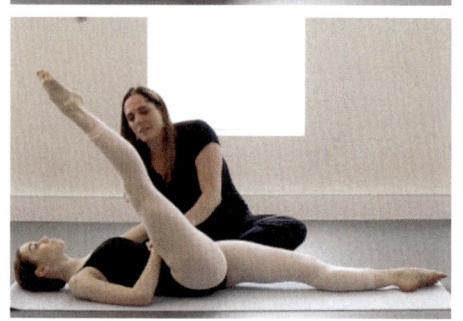

Placement at the Barre, with Fondu and Rise

This is a nice exercise to do with the foot on the barre to practice your pelvic control. When moving into standing many dancers tend to habitually tuck their pelvis under. We were often taught this position in an effort to activate turnout and deep core muscles, however in reality the tucked position encourages gripping of the outer gluteal muscles and inhibits the deep spinal stabilisers. This exercise helps you practice your deep back control and pelvic stability in standing, combined with the placement of the leg in front.

Level 1:
- Face towards the barre and place one foot onto it. You want to find a comfortable position, so try not to avoid the bony parts of your ankle.
- You may like to place a folded yoga mat or towel over the barre to make it more comfortable.
- Keep the spine in neutral and lift and lengthen the side waist.
- Make sure your deep back muscles are activated to support your neutral spine position and your deep rotators on your standing leg are gently activated to maintain your turnout.
- Spend a few moments connecting to the feeling of rotation of the leg on the barre, as well as the standing leg, and just breathe.
- Feel the expansion and collection of through the rib cage, and your connection to your diaphragm and pelvic floor.
- If you feel any tension or pulling down the leg or in the front of the hip, go back and try an appropriate mobiliser to release.

Level 2:
- Once you have established good placement in this position, slowly fondu on the supporting leg, making sure you're keeping lifted through the lumbar spine, and relaxed in the upper body.
- Make sure to keep the pelvis and ribcage square to the barre.
- Straighten the supporting leg, then slowly rise, making sure the hips stay square and you are gently lifted through the low back.
- You can place one hand on the barre for balance initially, or try with your arms in first, on your hips or just relaxed down.

Level 3:
- Once you feel confident with your placement try increasing the speed and progress to repeated fondu/relevé on one leg.
- Try performing this exercise side on to a mirror to observe your spinal control.
- Make sure not to sit into the supporting hip or tuck the tail under.

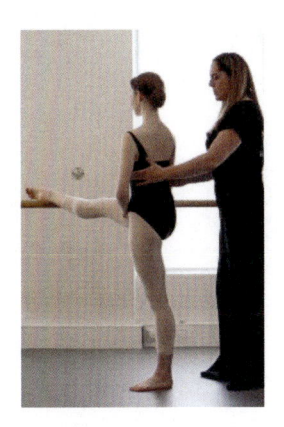

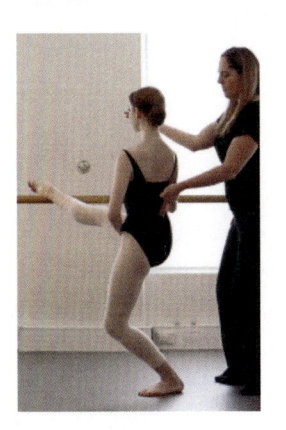

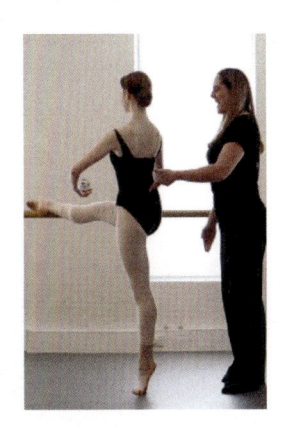

Notes:

Adage in Class

Ironically, once you get to performing your adage in class, you want to let go of thinking of all the specific muscles and elements that we have been working on. Try to feel fluidity of movement, and a light quality to your movement, like your leg is being held by someone other than you. The work that you have done in the rest of the program will start to shine through when you relax and work with the music.

If dancers try to control their adage too much it can become very stiff and wooden. This also contributes to a lot of the excessive contraction and loading that dancers feel around the hips when working en l'air. If you are to focus on anything, remember to breathe, to connect with the deepest sense of core stability, and generate every movement from your centre.

It may help to do some gentle hip mobilisers before working on your adage, but make sure not to hang out in any deep hip flexor stretches as this will inhibit the very muscles you need to use.

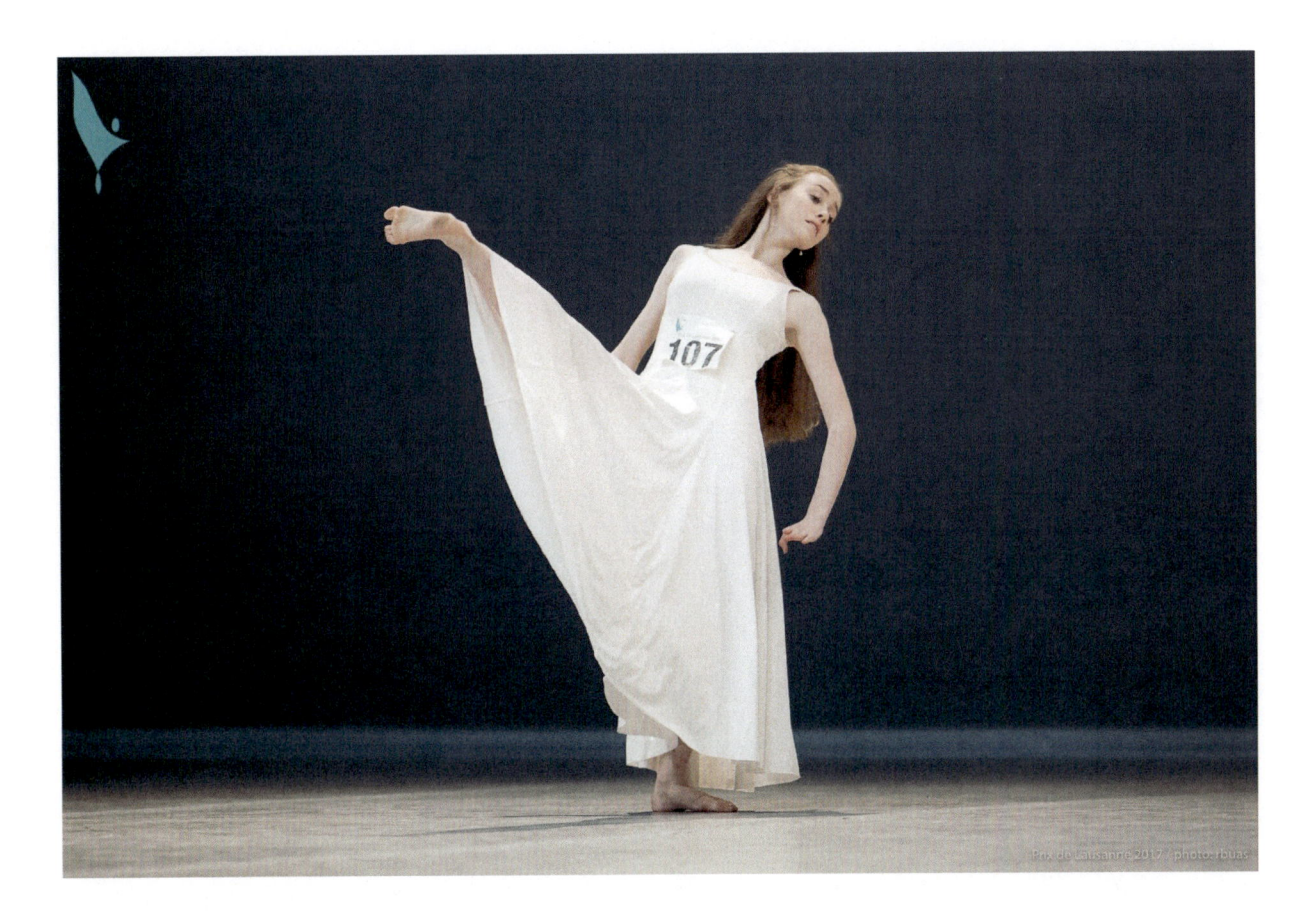

Putting Together Your Program

Once you have worked your way through the program and are starting to discover which parts of the program are important for you, it is important to organise a set program for you to work on. Always start from the beginning, from the mobilise section. Even if you have pretty good range it is a good idea to do the mobilisation exercises for at least 2 weeks to ensure that your range is free in all directions. See if you can work out a program that you will follow for at least 1-2 weeks, before adding in additional exercises. Each dancer needs to work on different elements, however a suggested guideline is outlined below.

Program 1	M	T	W	T	F	S	S
6 D Breathing							
Thoracic Mobilisers							
Hip Flexor Mobilisers							
Tucks and Tilts Sequence							
Trigger Point Releases with a Ball							
Cupping for Upper and Lower Legs							

Program 2	M	T	W	T	F	S	S
6 D Breathing							
Thoracic Mobilisers							
Hip Flexor Mobilisers							
Tucks and Tilts Sequence							
Trigger Point Releases with a Ball							
Cupping for Upper and Lower Legs							
4 Point Sit Backs							
Cushion Squeezes							
QF Heel Squeeze							

Program 3	M	T	W	T	F	S	S
6 D Breathing							
Thoracic Mobilisers							
Hip Flexor Mobilisers							
Tucks and Tilts Sequence							
Trigger Point Releases with a Ball							
4 Point Sit Backs							
Cushion Squeezes							
QF Heel Squeeze							
Iliacus Suck							
Turnout with Foot on the Wall							

Program 4	M	T	W	T	F	S	S
6 D Breathing							
Thoracic Mobilisers							
Hip Flexor Mobilisers							
Tucks and Tilts Sequence							
Waiter Bow							
Cushion Squeezes - with Leg Extension							
4 Point Turnout with Endurance							
Cushion Squeezes with Oblique Curl							
Turnout with Foot on the Wall							
Standing Iliacus Suck							
Adult Crawling Sequence							

Program 5	M	T	W	T	F	S	S
Hip Flexor Mobilisers							
Trigger Point Releases with Ball							
Tucks and Tilts Sequence							
Hamstring Mobilisers							
Waiter Bow							
Cushion Squeezes - with Leg Extension							
4 Point Turnout with Endurance							
Turnout with Foot on the Wall							
Standing Iliacus Suck							
Adult Crawling Sequence							
QF Transfer with Port de Bras							
Développé Devant in Lying							

Program 6	M	T	W	T	F	S	S
Hip Flexor Mobilisers							
Tucks and Tilts Sequence							
Hamstring Mobilisers							
Waiter Bow							
4 Point Turnout with Endurance							
Turnout with Foot on the Wall							
Standing Iliacus Suck							
Adult Crawling Sequence							
QF Transfer with Port de Bras							
Développé Devant in Lying							
Placement at the Barre with Fondu & Rise							

Acknowledgements

Thank you so much to every single client I have ever worked with. Your uniqueness, challenges and feedback have helped me hone our programs to be the most effective and efficient way of dealing with common issues, with enough customisation to ensure great results for everyone.

Huge thanks must also go to the hundreds of dance teachers worldwide who have attended my Teacher Training courses, and given such positive feedback on the application of these programs. I thrive off the feedback you give me and and your infectious enthusiasm inspires me to keep on giving.

Lisa xx

To gain access to the online video course that is the companion to this book please visit www.theballetblog.com. This course has videos of all of the exercises in much greater detail, as well as access to a bonus video and other features.

Related Resources

A New Approach to Core Stability

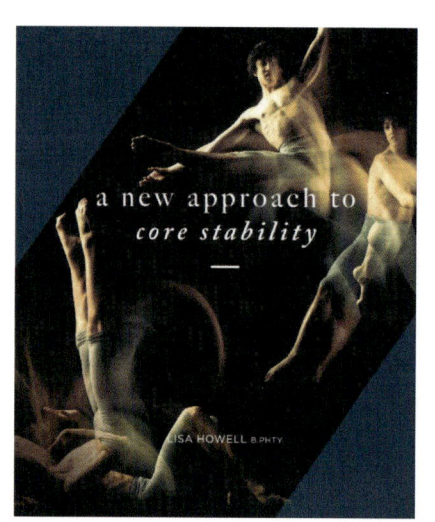

This book on "core stability" is based on evidence based medicine, and years of clinical experience, as well as the authors own journey with back pain. After being frustrated by the lack of resources that explained exactly what "core stability" is all about, and suffering back pain unnecessarily for years herself. She wanted to help everyone learn the secrets to get rid of constant nagging, and often excruciating back pain, and also be able to retrain their spine to be able to perform again at a high level, whether that be into deep back bends in yoga, running up stairs, managing 18 holes of gold or a 4 hour shopping expedition. This program demystifies the specifics of core stability that are essential in mastering control of your true core, and is essential to a full recovery from back pain, and has the added benefit of better performance of most sporting activities as well!

Front Splits Fast

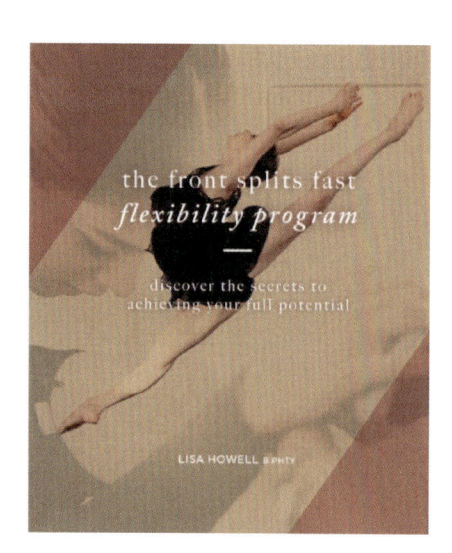

The Front Splits Fast Flexibility Program is a revolutionary program that is guaranteed to change how you think about flexibility forever! This exciting program translates techniques used by therapists into an easy to use program that you can work on at home to achieve instant and lasting changes in your flexibility. This program goes far beyond stretching, and is so much more effective than spending hours tugging at your muscles, trying to make them "longer". Cruise past your old limitations by learning secret techniques to mobilise your nervous system and release fascial tension (both of which can dramatically alter you flexibility). The program is presented in an easy to use format with detailed explanations of all of the exercises. This is a fantastic resource for anyone interested in increasing their mobility into the front splits!

To purchase these resources visit our website: https://www.theballetblog.com/

Made in the USA
Lexington, KY
04 April 2019